WHAT OTHER HEALTH CARE
PROFESSION...
THIS EXTRA...

D0596380

"*Remarkably comp...   e
Officer who cares fo...*"

- **William Jensen, M.D.**
Program Director
Dept. of Internal Medicine
Santa Clara Valley Medical Center

"*A great OB-GYN summary, <u>a real time-saver</u>... an excellent reference for the non-Spanish speaking professional.*"

- **David Plourd, M.D.**
Senior Staff Physician
Dept. of Obstetrics & Gynecology
Santa Clara Valley Medical Center

"*<u>Quick and to the point</u>. A neat little guide for the health care provider - from triage nurses to paramedics.*"

- **Gloria Jennings, M.U.C.**
Medical Unit Clerk
Dept. of Emergency Medicine
Santa Clara Valley Medical Center

"*Thank goodness... Small enough to fit into my scrub pocket and <u>useful enough to carry everywhere</u>.*"

- **Eric Dummel, M.D.**
Medical Resident
Dept. of Internal Medicine
Kaiser Hospital, San Francisco

With this guide you won't need to speak Spanish to understand the responses to critical questions!

SURVIVAL SPANISH

A POCKET GUIDE FOR THE MEDICAL PROFESSIONAL

2ND EDITION

T. P. SKAARUP, M.D.

PARA MI ESPOSA, PAULA

Survival Spanish/T.P. Skaarup
Grey's Notes
P.O. Box 2005
Elk Grove, CA   95759-2005

10 9 8 7 6 5 4 3 2

Library of Congress Catalog Card Number: 91-061505
ISBN 1-879671-01-8

Text was typeset in Palatino 6-12 pt., Lithos 12-24 pt., & Lithos Black 6-12 pt., 600 DPI. Spiral binding only available on non-promotional release.

And yes Eric, I did type every stinking word in this book. *tps*

PRINTED IN THE UNITED STATES OF AMERICA

INTRODUCTION TO THE FIRST EDITION

"¿Le corren las narices?" The patient sat dumb-struck, holding the infant in her arms. Her face formed an expression as if to say, "do I trust this doctor with my child?" I knew that something had gone wrong...

Earlier that day I sensed something was out of whack when I discovered all four copies of a comprehensive Spanish phrase book on the shelf of our hospital library. Valley Medical Center serves a large Hispanic population and I thought it unusual, if not improbable, that all four copies were on the shelf and not in use on the wards and clinics.

I'd jeered at the Translator in Peds clinic that morning, "With my bad Spanish and this book... you'll be out of a job!" He glanced first at me, then the phrase book, and sneered – then was suddenly gone, the sound of his beeper trailing in the distance. "Adiós amigo. For good." I turned to the 'patients-to-be-seen' board with nine patients waiting and six spoke only Spanish.

By now I had cared for Spanish speaking patients for just over two years. Mostly with the aid of a Spanish translator and my pocket collection of phrases I could muddle through a medical history. Today would be different. I had the "comprehensive" guide. But now something was going wrong...

I repeated the phrase again, *"¿Le corren las narices?"* and received a familiar blank stare. I pointed to the phrase in the book as I read it, hoping the patient could follow along and understand. She motioned that she could not read. I called for the Spanish translator.

....

"¿Le corren las narices?" roughly translates to "do your nostrils run?" or "does your nose race?" I might have well been asking, "Is your refrigerator running? - better go catch it!" The phrase, **"runny** nose," is an American colloquialism. It makes little or no sense translated literally into another language. This encounter did little to stimulate confidence in the American health care system.

It was more or less at that moment that I decided to undertake the massive task of compiling, typing, editing, and field-testing a list of handy and useful phrases in medical Spanish.

ACKNOWLEDGEMENTS AND ORIGINS

I began collecting Spanish phrases while a medical student at the University of Southern California School of Medicine, USC-LAC Medical Center in Los Angeles, California. The first medical Spanish I ever learned center around phlebotomy (the art of drawing blood). I progressed to simple medical rounds questions such as, "pain?" (*¿dolor?*) , "better?" (*¿mejor?*) and "where?" (*¿dónde?*). During this time, I kept a growing collection of Spanish phrases on a series of 3x5" cards in the front pocket of my scrubs.

During my senior year, I published a short "Survival Guide" for the USC-LAC Medical Center. Among other things, this guide included twelve pages of medical Spanish. Basically, the pages were a typewritten transcript of phrases in my pocket. These pages served as the primal origins of this book - and also helped name this "pocket guide."

As I undertook this project, I began scribbling furiously any time the Spanish translator was around. I collected phrase-lists kept on clinic walls or under plastic desk covers at patient registration counters. I asked physicians & nurses about their favorite Spanish phrases. All in all, what you have in your hands (the second edition) represents about one-thousand hours of work.

The majority of the historical and review-of-systems comes from an outline (provided in the first section of this book) which I used as a medical student.

THANKS TO:
- *Virginia Amaya*, Texan by birth but raised in San Jose, California so that makes her okay
- *Alejandro Chavarria*, the Nicaragüan, a man of peace through both actions and words
- *Roberta Cunningham*, the bombshell from South America, whose missionary family lived in Argentina, Bolivia, and Chile and who treats all Interns as 'mi corazón'
- *Gloria Perez*, who learned Spanish on the streets of San Jose, California, and runs amok in the ER of Valley Med
- *Miriam Larsen*, from Mexico City, Mexico, the red hot chile pepper who routinely rescues us *gringos* in clinic
- *Sergio Aldan*, the Mexican physician who helped me with the colloquial dictionary and interpreted the culture for me
- *Ricardo "Ronx" Ronquillo*, a Stanford medical student (and darned snappy dresser) for his help in proof-reading.
- *Robert Hofkins*, retired police officer, would-be baseball great, for his collection of police phrases.

TABLE OF CONTENTS

FEEDBACK...

Thank you for your response to the first edition. As you've suggested, I've modified many of the sections, completely rewriting some, adding others. I hope you find changes along with the addition of a 6,500 entry dictionary useful.

So now I call on you again - I would like to expand this volume even more! I would enjoy your input - from spelling to content, punctuation to praises, criticism to phrases. Most especially though, I want to know how I can modify this book to be more useful. Send me phrases! I am looking for phrases to round off the edges of this humble book, *especially phrases dealing with nursing, nutrition, paramedic, physical therapy, police, chiropractic, social work, medical and surgical sub-specialty settings.* Feel free to write me through my publisher (the address is listed on the copyright notice). I'm not promising I can answer every letter, but be assured, I read every letter I receive.

PHRASING OF QUESTIONS
You don't have to speak Spanish to understand the answers to the phrases in this book. I have attempted to phrase my questions in such a manner that they may be answered with either a *"yes,"* a *"no,"* a *number,* or a *date.* When this is not possible, I've tried to include a list of potential replies. If your patient replies too rapidly or answers with a reply other than "yes" or "no," try the following:

• **Please answer "yes" or "no" to my questions...**	Por favor conteste "si" o "no" a mis preguntas...
• **Please answer my questions slowly...**	Por favor conteste mis preguntas despacio...
• **Not so fast...**	¡No tan rápido!
• **I need you to help me understand you...**	Yo necesito que usted me ayude a comprenderlo,-a
• **Write down the date...**	Escriba la fecha...
• **Write down the number...**	Escriba el numero...

Remember, to *"Hablar en gringo"* is "to speak in nonsense."

THE PAST MEDICAL HISTORY

- **HISTORY & PHYSICAL OUTLINE**
- **PATIENT REGISTRATION**
- **PAST MEDICAL HISTORY**
  CHILDHOOD ILLNESSES
  ADULT ILLNESSES/HOSPITALIZATIONS
  SURGERIES/ACCIDENTS
  SOCIAL HABITS
  ILLEGAL DRUGS
- **FAMILY HISTORY**
- **MEDICATION HISTORY**

- As an organization tool, I've included a standard Medical History & Physical Exam outline which I used as a medical student. I've attempted to translate these historical points into a series of "yes" or "no" questions. When a simple "yes" or "no" is not possible, I've provided an alternate list from which to choose a suitable response.

- The History and Physical outline provided may also serve as a format for dictating reports or as a guideline for a formal written presentation.

MEDICAL HISTORY

IDENTIFYING DATA/CHIEF COMPLAINT:
Age, race, sex, chief complaint and duration of complaint

HISTORY OF PRESENT ILLNESS:
1. Overview of patients health
2. Characterize the patients current problems in depth. Create a
   continuous time-stream until the present. Relate symptoms to
   relevant past history, personal history, family history, prescribed drugs, consultations, test results, etc. Keep it brief and
   to the point. Use the PQRST format for each symptom: **P:**
   (**p**rovocative/**p**alliative), **Q:** (**q**uality/**q**uantity), **R:** (radia-
   tion/location), **S:** (**s** everity/debility), **T:** (time associa-
   tions/duration)
3. Pertinent ROS (pertinent positives and negatives).

PAST MEDICAL HISTORY:
1. Medical: (A) Childhood diseases (B) Adult medical illnesses
   (e.g. HTN, CAD, DM)
2. Surgical/Fractures
3. Hospitalizations/Accidents
4. Prescribed drugs, Over the counter drugs
5. Allergies and Immunizations *(Pediatrics Only):* Number of
   adults living at home, any sick contacts (children or adults) at
   home.
6. HEADSS *(Adolecents)*: Home Life, Education Level, Activities,
   Drug Use, Sexual Activity, Suicide Idealization or Attempts
7. Habits: Alcohol (EtOH), Tobacco, IV Drug Abuse (IVDA)
8. Birth History *(Pediatrics only):* Maternal **G:**(total pregnancies)
   P:(full term, pre-term, abortions, living), Duration of Labor,
   Caesarean section (C/S) or Vaginal Delivery (NSVD), Where
   born, Gestational Age, Illness During Pregnancy,
   Complications. How many days in hospital before discharge
   for mother and infant.
9. Developmental History *(Pediatrics Only):* Raises Head, Crawl,
   Eye-to-Eye contact, Cruise, Social Smile, Walk, Lifts from
   Prone, Climb Stairs, Sits alone, Down Stairs

FAMILY HISTORY:
1. Age, health or parents, siblings, children, spouse
2. MI, DM, HTN, TB, Stroke, Arthritis, CA, EtOH, Emotional
   problems. Any unusual illness or early deaths
3. Effect of patient's illness on family

REVIEW OF SYSTEMS (R.O.S.)

GENERAL General state of health, recent changes in weight, appetite, fevers, chills, nausea, emesis, colds, sore throat, or night sweats.

SKIN rashes, chronic problems, tattoos, scars.

HEENT *HEAD*: headache, injury *EYE*: acuity, diplopia, blurring, trauma, pain, discharge, glasses *EAR*: changes in hearing, tinnitus, vertigo, pain, discharge *NOSE*: discharges, nosebleeds, trauma, blockage *MOUTH*: bleeding gums, dental caries, tongue changes, difficulty chewing *THROAT*: difficulty swallowing, hoarseness, pain *NECK*: lumps, swollen glands, thyroid, problems, pain.

PULMONARY cough, sputum, hemoptysis, shortness of breath (SOB) +/- wheezing, shortness of breath on exertion (SOBOE), smoking, chest pain, last CXR (normal/abnormal).

CARDIAC chest pain, palpitations, shortness of breath (SOB), shortness of breath on exertion (SOBOE), paroxysmal noctunal dyspnea (PND), orthopnea, edema or swelling of ankles (SOA), murmurs, hypertension (HTN), past heart attacks (MI).

BREASTS pain, discharge, trauma, lumps .

GASTROINTESTINAL weight changes, pain, changes in appetite, nausea/vomiting, diarrhea/constipation, melena, hematochezia, hematemesis, hemorrhoids, clay colored stools, jaundice/hepatitis, gall bladder disease, excessive gas, burping, or excessive flatus.

GENITO-URINARY dysuria, frequency, urgency, nocturia, hesitancy, hematuria, discharges, history of STDs, sexual function prob. FEMALE ONLY: menarche age, menstrual triad (cycle, duration, dysmenorrhea) vaginal discharge (color, amount, odor, consistency, pain, itching), number of pregnancies, number of deliveries, number of abortions, number of children living, problem during delivery, last PAP (date & result), menopausal symptoms.

HEMATOLOGICAL history of anemia (specify), easy bruising, persisting bleeding, HIV antibody test.

ENDOCRINE thyroid problems (hot/cold intolerance), easily fatigued, history of polyuria/polydipsia, diabetes, other.

MUSCULOSKELETAL joint pains, redness, swelling, decreased function, myalgia, back pain, other musculoskeletal symptoms.

NEUROPSYCHIATRIC dizziness, vertigo, syncope, seizures, parasthesias, tremors, changes in memory, speech problems, emotional problems (depression, suicide, anxiety, history of past psychiatric care).

PHYSICAL EXAMINATION (P.E.)

GENERAL: appearance, race, state of nutrition, physique (habitus), apparent age, sign of acute or chronic distress, activity level, alertness, orientation, breathing pattern, pallor, position of patient (e.g. "resting on gurney")

VITAL SIGNS: BP, pulse, temperature, respiratory rate, height, weight, oxygen saturation

SKIN: color, moisture, temperature, turgor, hair patterns, lesions, tattoos, rashes, surgical wounds, acute or chronic changes.

HEENT: *HEAD:* signs of trauma, masses, tenderness, scalp, bruit *EARS:* gross hearing, external, pinna, canal, TM, landmarks, mobility, light reflex, Weber, Renne *EYES:* acuity, visual fields, EOM, conjunctivae, sclera, limbus, corneal reflex, PERRL, disc, cup, artery, vein, A/V ratio, silver wiring *NOSE:* patency, septum intact, mucosa (signs of inflammation), discharge *SINUSES:* palp for tenderness, frontal, mastoid, maxillary, transillumination (prn) *MOUTH:* inspection of lips, tongue, mucosa, teeth, caries, oral hygeine *THROAT:* pharynx, tonsils, uvular deviation, gag reflex *NECK:* supple, range of motion (ROM), thyroid exam, trachea position, carotid pulse, bruits, lymph node palpation, jugular venous distension (JVD)

PULMONARY: IPPA: configuration, resp. movements, rate, pattern, cyanosis, clubbing; fremitus, crepitus, pleural rub; lung field resonance, diaphragm excursion; type of breath sounds, (bronchial, egophony, bronchophony, whispered pectoriloquy, wheeze), crackles, ronchi, pleural rubs,

CARDIAC: IPPA: cyanosis, clubbing, pallor, JVD, edema, precordial activity (visible lifts and heaves); PMI, thrills, HJR; position of apex; valve areas (mitral, tricuspid, aortic, pulmonic), S1/S2, S2 split (inspiratory), S3 or S4 "gallops," murmurs

BREAST: symmetry, masses, nipple discharge, skin changes, axillary nodes, supraclavicular & infraclavicular nodes

ABDOMEN: AIPP: bowel sounds; contour, movements, hair patterns, umbilicus, scars, venous distention; tenderness (direct and rebound), masses, spleen, liver; borders of spleen, borders of liver, masses, ascites

RECTAL: external, sphincter tone, masses, prostate exam, stool occult blood, tags, fissures, hemorrhoids, warts

GENITALIA: *MALE:* meatus, penis, scrotum, testes, hernia, hydrocele; *FEMALE:* external genitalia, vagina, cervix, uterus, adnexae, rectovaginal, cervical motion tenderness

VASCULAR: (rate, rhythm, intensity) carotid, radial, brachial, femoral, popliteal, post tibial, dorsalis pedis

NODES: cervical, suboccipital, pre & post auricular, axillary, supraclavicular, epitrochlear, inguinal

EXTREMITIES & MUSCULOSKELETAL:

GENERAL: nails, clubbing, edema, skin changes, hair changes, varicosities;

JOINTS: ROM, redness, swelling, hotness, decreased function, abnormal configuration;

BACK: configuration (kyphosis, scoliosis, lumbardosis), Adam's (scoliosis) test, costo-vertebral angle tenderness (CVAT)

NEUROLOGICAL:

CRANIAL NERVES: See below

MOTOR: walk heel-to-toe, walk toe-to-toe, hop in place, rise from sitting, arms straight ahead (30 sec), arms above head (30 sec), press forward (winging), two finger grip, Rhomberg (eyes open & closed) ;

SENSORY: pain (pin prick), temperature, light touch, vibration, position, discriminative sensations, stereognosis, number recognition, 2-point discrimination, point localization, extinction;

DTR'S: Biceps (C5-6), Triceps (C6-8), Brachioradialis (C5-6), Knee (L2-4), Abdominal (T8-12), Ankle/Gastroc. (S1-2), Plantar (L4-S2), Masseter (V), Trapezius (XI)

MENTAL STATUS: Appearance & behavior; Awake/Alert; Speech (vocabulary, quantity, coherence); Mood; Perceptions (illusions, hallucinations); Orientation X 4 (person, place, time, purpose); Thinking (content, abstraction, recent and remote memory)

CRANIAL NERVES
I	Smell (primary scents) or by patient report
II	Vision (direct/ concentual reflexes)
III	EOM (all except...)
IV	EOM (sup. oblique)
VI	EOM (abducens)
V	Sensory (facial: V1-ophthalmic, V2-maxillary, V3-mandibular) if abnormal, test hot/cold, light touch, and corneal. Motor (masseter, temporal)
VII	Facial expression, platysmus, raise eyebrow, frown, smile, close eyes tight, show upper, lower teeth, puff out cheeks
VIII	Hearing, whisper, Webber and if indicated, Renne
IX/X	Gag reflex, midline uvula
XI	Trapezius and sternocleidomastoid
XII	Protrude tongue midline

OPENING LINES

I am just learning to speak Spanish...	*Yo estoy apenas aprendiendo a hablar Español...*
I don't speak good Spanish...	*No hablo muy bien español...*
My Spanish is very poor	*Mi español es muy pobre*
I speak very little Spanish	*Yo hablo muy poco español*
I need you to help me to understand	*You necesito que usted me ayude a comprenderlo,-a*
I don't speak Spanish	*Yo no hablo español*
Speak slowly, please	*Hable despacio, por favor*
I speak a little Spanish	*Yo hablo un poco de español*
I'm reading from a list of questions...	*Estoy leyendo de un questionario varias preguntas...*
That I need to know about you	*Que necesito saber de usted*
Please answer "yes" or "no" to my questions...	**Por favor conteste "si" o "no" a mis preguntas...**
Please answer my questions slowly...	**Por favor conteste mis preguntas despacio...**
Understand (me)?	*¿(Me) Entiende?*
If you can, answer ...	*Si puede, conteste ...*
...with "yes" or "no"	*...con "sí" o "no"*
...in a fashion that I can understand	*...de modo que pueda entenderle*
...in a more precise fashion	*...de modo más preciso*
Give me only the...	*Déme solamente el/la...*
...name/number	*...nombre/número*
...date/time	*...fecha/hora*
Write down the number...	*Escriba el numero...*
Write down the date...	*Escriba la fecha...*
Write down the name...	*Escriba el nombre...*
How do you spell it?	*¿Cómo se deletrea?*

REGISTRATION

Do you need to see a doctor?	*¿Necesita ver a un doctor/ médico?*
Do you have a friend who speaks English (with you)?	*¿Tiene un amigo que habla ingles (con usted)?*
Do you have your (blue), (green), (red), (yellow) card?	*¿Tiene su tarjeta (azul), (verde), (roja), (amarilla)?*
Have you been here before (in the past __ years)? Recently?	*¿Ha venido aquí antes (en el pasado __ años)? ¿Reciente- mente?*
Follow the yellow/ blue/ black/ white line on the floor...	*Siga la linea anarilla/ azul/ negro/ blanco en el suelo...*
Come with me...	*Venga conmigo...*

REGISTRATION

Who is the patient?	*¿Quién es el paciente?*
What is the name of the patient?	*¿Cuál es el nombre del paciente?*
"How are you called?" [name]	*¿Cómo se llama? [nombre]*
What is your name?	*¿Cuál es su nombre?*
What is your...	*¿Cuál es su...*
...First Name?	*...Primer Nombre?*
...Initial?	*...Inicial?*
...Last Name?	*...Apellido?*
...Nick Name	*...Apodar/Sobrenombre*
What is your address?	*¿Cuál es su dirección?*
What is your ZIP-Code?	*¿Cuál es su zona postal?*
What is your telephone number?	*¿Cuál es su número de teléfono?*
Have you been going to clinic? Which clinic?	*¿Ha venido a la clinica? ¿Cuál clinica?*

INSURANCE

What is your social security number?	*¿Cuál es su número de seguro social?*
Do you have work ?	*¿Tiene trabajo?*
What is the name of your employer?	*¿Cuál es el nombre de su empleador?*
Do you have insurance?	*¿Tiene seguro?*
What is your insurance company?	*¿Cuál es su compañia de seguro?*
Have you...	*¿Tiene...*
...Medicare/Medi-Cal?	*...Medicare/Medi-Cal?*
...Blue Cross/Blue Shield?	*...Cruz Azul/Escudo Azul?*
...Kaiser?	*...de Kaiser?*

PERSONAL/SOCIAL

How many years do you have (age)?	¿Cuándo años tiene (edad)?
What is your age?	¿Qué edad tiene?
How much do you weigh (in pounds)?	¿Cuanto pesa (en libras)?
Height (in feet)?	¿Estatura (en pies)?
Date of birth?	¿Fecha de nacimiento?
Are you married?	¿Es usted casado?
...Single	...Soltero
...Divorced	...Divorciado
...Separated	...Separado
...Widow/Widower	...Viudo/Viuda
You live with your spouse?	¿Vive usted con su esposa/ esposo?
How many years of education do you have?	¿Cuántos años de educación tiene?
What is your religion?	¿Cuál es su religión?
How long have you lived in the United States (of America)?	¿Cuánto tiempo ha vivido en los Estados Unidos (de América)?
Are you an American citizen?	¿Es ciudadano Americano?
Of what country are you?	¿De qué país es usted?
Where were you born?	¿Dónde nació?

FORMS

Fill (out) the forms	Llene los formularios
Fill out this form...	Llene ésta forma...
Please fill out this form...	Favor de llenar esta forma
Read it and sign it... please	Léala y fírmela... por favor
Sign here, please...	Firme aquí, por favor...
Sign the authorization...	Firme la autorización:
Write your address	Escriba su dirección.

PAST MEDICAL HISTORY (BRIEF)

CHILDHOOD ILLNESSES

Do you have or have you had (at any time)...?	*¿Tiene o ha tenido (alguna vez)...?*
Cancer	*Cáncer*
Chicken Pox	*Varicela, Viruelas Locas*
Asthma	*Asma*
Bleeding Tendency	*Tendencia a Sangrar*
Diabetes	*Diabetes*
Diptheria	*Difteria*
Epilepsy	*Epilepsia*
Fractures	*Fracturas*
Leukemia	*Leucemia*
Measles	*Sarampion*
Mumps	*Paperas*
German Measles	*Rubéola*
Rheumatic Fever	*Fiebre reumática*
Heart Disease	*Enfermedades de Corazón*
Small Pox	*Viruelas*
Seizures	*Convulsiones*
Scarlet Fever	*Escarlatina*
Tumors	*Tumors*
Typhus	*Tifus*
Typhoid	*Tifoidea*
Ulcer	*Ulcera*
Whooping Cough	*Tos Ferina*

ADULT ILLNESSES*

Do you have or have you had (at any time)...?	*¿Tiene o ha tenido (alguna vez)...?*
...Any Serious Illness?	*...Alguna Enfermedad Seria?*
...Been Hospitalized?	*...Ha Sido Hopitalizadao?*
When? In which hospital?	*¿Cuándo? ¿En cuál hospital?*
Write down the date/the name of the hospital...	*Escriba la fecha/el nombre del hospital...*
Have you had a transfusion (infusion) of blood?	*¿Ha tenido una tranfusion (infusion) de sangre?*

* Please refer to Vocabulary section "Symptoms/Chief Compaints" for an exhaustive list of adult illnesses.

SURGERIES/ACCIDENTS

Have you had (any)…?	*¿Ha tenido (algunas)…?*
…Operations? For what?	…Operaciónes? ¿De qué?
…They took out your tonsils?	…¿Le sacaron las amígdala/ glandulas salivares?
…They took out your appendix?	…¿Le sacaron la apéndice?
…They took out your uterus?	…¿Le sacaron matriz?
…They took out the ovaries?	…¿Le sacaron los ovarios?
…They took out your gall baldder?	…¿Le sacaron su véscícula (biliar)?
…Major accidents	…Accidentes graves
…Broken a bone	…Se ha quebrado un hueso
…Fractures	…Fracturas
…Lost conciousness	…Ha pérdido el conocimiento
…Injury or concussion	…Daño o concusiones cerebrales

SOCIAL HABITS

Smoke?	¿Fuma?
How many packs a day (week)?	¿Cuántos cajillas (paquetes) al dia (por semana)?
Drink?	¿Toma?
Every day? ("all the days")	¿Todos los días?
How many a day?	¿Cuántas al dia?
How many bottles a day (week)?	¿Cuántas botellas al dia (semana)?
…Alcohol	…Alcohol
…Beer	…Cerveza
…Wine	…Vino "Vee-No"
…Whiskey	…Whiskey "We-Ski"

ILLEGAL DRUGS

Do you use or have you used (at any time)…?	*¿Usa o ha usado (alguna vez)…?*
…Intravenous Drugs	…Drogas Intravenosas
…Cocaine	…Cocaína
…Crack	…Crac ("Crak")
…Heroin	…Heroína
…Marijuana	…Marijuana
…Methadone	…Metadona
…Opium	…Opio
…Or Any Others Drug	…O Alguna Otra Droga

FAMILY HISTORY

Anyone in your family have or every had illnesses of...?

¿Alguno de su familia estuvo o ha estado enfermo de...?

...Arthritis	...Artritis
...Asthma	...Asma
...Bleeding Tendency	...Tendencia a Sangrar
...Cancer (CA)	...Cáncer
...Diabetes (DM)	...Diabetes
...Emphysema	...Enfisema
...Epilepsy	...Epilepsia
...Gout	...Gota
...Heart Attack (MI)	...Ataque al Corazón
...Heart Disease	...Enfermedades de Corazón
...Heart Failure	...Falla Cardiaca
...Hemophilia	...Hemofilia
...High Blood Pressure (HTN)	...Alta Presión
...Insanity	...Locura
...Psychosis	...Psicosis
...Seizures	...Convulsiones/Ataques
...Stroke	...Apoplejía/Derrame Cerebral
...Suicide	...Suicidio
...Tuberculosis (TB)	...Tuberculosis

Do you have brothers & sisters?	¿Tiene hermanos?
Are your parents living?	¿Están vivos sus padres?
Are your parents dead?	¿Están muertos sus padres?
How did your mother/father/ sister/brother die?	¿Cómo murió su madre/ padre/hermana/hermano?
Do you have any children?	¿Tiene algunas hijos/niños?

(Please see "Relatives" in the Vocabulary Section for a complete list of family members.)

Wife	Esposa	Husband	Esposo
Mother	Madre/Mamá	Father	Padre/Papá
Sister	Hermana	Brother	Hermano
Daughter/ Son	Hija/ Hijo	Aunt/Uncle	Tía/Tío
Grandmother	Abuela	Grandfather	Abuelo
Granddaughter	Nieta	Grandson	Nieto
Cousin (F/M)	Prima/Primo	Child-Girl/Boy	Niña/Niño
Woman/Man	Mujer/Hombre		

MEDICATION HISTORY

What medicines have you been taking?	*¿Qué medicinas ha estado tomando?*
What medicines do you have to take?	*¿Qué medicinas tiene que tomar?*
Do you have your medicines with you?	*¿Tiene sus medicinas con usted?*
What are the names of your medicines?	*¿Cuáles son los nombres de sus medicinas?*
You take medicines?	*¿Toma medicinas…?*
…Aspirin/Tylenol	*…Aspirina/Tylenol*
…Iron/Vitamins	*…Hierro/Vitaminas*
…Liquid/Drops	*…Liquido/Gotas*

Do you have to take medicines for…?	*¿Tiene usted que tomar medicinas para…?*
…the Heart	*… el Corazón*
…the Liver	*… el Hígado*
…the Kidney	*…los Riñones*
…the Nerves	*…los Nervios*
…to Sleep	*…Dormir*
…Pain	*…Dolor*
…Diabetes/Inject Insulin?	*…Diabetes/Inyectar Insulina?*
How many (times) a day?	*¿Cuántas (veces) al día?*

Are you allergic to medicines or foods?	*¿Es alérgica a medicinas o comidas/almientos?*
Do you have allergies to medicines or foods?	*¿Tiene alérgias a medicinas o comidas/almientos?*

Do you have an allergy to…?	*¿Tiene alérgia a…?*
…Penicillin	*…Penicilina*
…Aspirin	*…Aspirina*
…Sulfa Drugs	*…Drogas "Sulfa"*
…Anesthesia	*…Anestesia*
…Antibiotics	*…Antibióticos*
…Foods	*…Comidas*
…Other Medicines	*…Otra Medicinas*
…Fish	*…Pescado*
…Seafood	*…Marisco*

THE REVIEW OF SYSTEMS

- CONSTITUTIONAL SYMPTOMS
- HEAD/EYES/EARS/NOSE/THROAT
- PULMONARY
- CARDIAC
- BREASTS
- GENITOURINARY
- GASTROINTESTINAL
- HEMATOLOGICAL
- ENDOCRINE
- MUSCULOSKELETAL
- SKIN
- NEUROPSYCHIATRIC
- MENSTRUAL
- SEXUAL HISTORY
- HIV SYMPTOMS

- It's been said that eighty percent of all medical diagnoses can be made based soley upon a careful and thorough history. Therefore, it's obvious that obtaining a good history is essential for rendering proper medical care.

- Additionally, a well performed medical history can help focus the physical examination and provide clues to specific diagnostic tests.

- Briefly, the "Review of Systems" is a body of questions used to create a database of information about a given patients health. Most, if not all, of the questions should be asked . It is not uncommon to have a patient state they are in "great shape," only to discover after some verbal poking and proding (i.e. the Review of Systems) that they are in great shape, except for a heart attack two years ago, the four abdominal surgeries for ulcers, and the two pills they have to take three times a day.

CONSTITUTIONAL SYMPTOMS General state of health, recent changes in weight, appetite, fevers, chills, nausea, emesis, colds, sore throat, dysuria, or night sweats

---

Have you been in good health recently?	*¿Ha estado en buena salud recientemente?*
Has your weight changed recently?	*¿Ha cambiado de peso recientemente?*
Have you lost weight recently?	*¿Ha perdido peso recientemente?*
Have you gained in weight?	*¿Ha aumentado de peso?*
How many pounds (more or less)?	*¿Cuántas libras (más o menos)?*
How is your appetite? Good or bad?	*¿Cómo esta su apetito? ¿Bueno o malo?*
Do you have fevers or chills?	*¿Tiene fiebre (calentura) o escalofríos?*
Do you have a cough? With phlegm?	*¿Tiene tos? ¿Con Flema?*
Do you have nausea or vomiting?	*¿Tiene náusea o vómitos?*
Do you have diarrhea or constipation?	*¿Tiene diarrea o estreñimiento?*
Have you a cold/flu?	*¿Está resfriado o tiene gripe?*
Do you have a sore throat?	*¿Tiene dolor de garganta?*
Do you have pain or burning at urination?	*¿Tiene dolor o ardor al orinar?*
Do you have sweats at night?	*¿Tiene sudores en la noche?*
Do you feel weak or tired?	*¿Se siente débil o cansado?*
Have you had a test for tuberculosis (on the skin)?	*¿Le han hecho una prueba de tuberculosis (en la piel)?*

Spanish Note: "Angina" is used in English to refer to chest pain. Angina in Spanish has two meanings. It refers to chest pain, but it can also be used to refer to a sore throat. So if your patient complains of severe angina (*anginas muy fuerte*), be sure of which pain your patient is complaining about. You wouldn't want to admit your patient to the Coronary Care Unit for a simple pharyngitis.

HEENT (HEAD, EARS, EYES, NOSE, THROAT): *HEAD*:
headache, injury *EYE*: acuity, diplopia, blurring, trauma, pain,
discharge/tearing, glasses *EAR*: changes in hearing, tinnitus,
vertigo, pain, discharge *NOSE*: discharges, trauma, blockage
MOUTH: bleeding gums, dental caries, tongue changes, difficulty chewing *THROAT*: difficulty swallowing, hoarseness, pain
NECK: lumps, swollen glands, thyroid, problems.

HEAD:

Do you have headaches?

Have you had injury to your head?

CABEZA:

¿Tiene dolores de cabeza?

¿Ha tenido heridas en la cabeza?

EYES:

Any problems with your vision?

Do you see double?

Do you have blurred vision (at times)?

Have you spots/stars in front of the eyes?

Do you have injury to your eyes?

Do you have eye pain?

Do you have glaucoma?

Do you have discharge from the eyes?

Do you have tearing in the eyes?

Do you have itching of the eyes?

Do you use glasses/lenses?

OJOS:

¿Algun problema con su vista/ visión?

¿Ve doble?

¿Tiene la vista borrosa (a veces)?

¿Ha tenido manchas/estrellas enfrente de los ojos?

¿Tiene heridas en los ojos?

¿Tiene dolores en los ojos?

¿Tiene glaucoma?

¿Le supuran los ojos? ¿Le sale pus por los ojos?

¿Tiene lagrimas en los ojos?

¿Tiene comezón de los ojos?

¿Usa (anteojos/gafas)/lentes?

EARS:

Any problems with your hearing?

Do you feel ringing in your ears?

Do you have discharge from the ears?

Do you have injury to your ears?

Do you have ear pain?

Do you feel dizzy or do you have vertigo?

OÍDOS:

¿Algun problema al oír?

¿Siente ruido/tintineo en los oídos?

¿Le supuran los oídos? ¿Le sale pus por los oídos?

¿Tiene heridas en los oídos?

¿Tiene dolores en los oídos?

¿Se siente mareado o tiene vértigo?

NOSE:

Have you injury to your nose?

Do you have a "runny nose"?

Have you a stuffy nose?

Have you nose bleeds?

Can you breath by nose (both sides)?

Problems with your sinuses (sinusitis)?

NARIZ:

¿Tiene heridas en la nariz?

¿Tiene catarro (en la nariz) o moquean/mocos?

¿Tiene la nariz tapada?

¿Le sangra la nariz?

¿Puede respirar por la nariz (dos lados)?

¿Problemas con los senos nasales (sinusitis)?

MOUTH:

Bleeding at the gums?

Any changes in your tongue?

Any difficulty chewing?

BOCA:

¿Le sangra la encilla?

¿Algun cambio en la lengua?

¿Algunas dificultades al mascar?

THROAT:

Have you difficulty swallowing?

Have you problems when swallowing?

Have you any hoarseness?

Are you hoarse?

Have you a sore throat?

GARGANTA:

¿Tiene dificultad al tragar?

¿Tiene problemas cuando traga?

¿Tiene algunas ronqueras?

¿Esta ronco?

¿Tiene dolor de garganta?

NECK:

Have you neck pain or feel stiff?

Any bumps/lumps in your neck?

Have you enlarged or inflamed glands?

Have you problems with the thyroid?

Noticed any swelling in the neck?

CUELLO:

¿Tiene dolor del cuello o siente el cuello tieso/duro?

¿Algunas bultos o bolitas en el cuello?

¿Tiene las glándula crecidas o inflamadas?

¿Tiene problemas con la tiroides?

¿Nota alguna inflamación/ hinchazón en el cuello?

Spanish Note: "Cerebro," the Spanish word for "brain," can also be used to refer to the posterior part of the head (occiput). If your patient complains of pain in the "cerebro," he may not be saying that his brain hurts, but rather it's the back of his head that's bothering him.

PULMONARY cough, sputum, hemoptysis, shortness of breath (SOB) (+/- wheezing), shortness of breath on exertion (SOBOE), smoking, chest pain, history of TB/pneumonia, last CXR (normal/abnormal)

Any problems with the lungs?	*¿Algunas problemas con los pulmones?*
Have a cold or have you the flu?	*¿Está resfriado o tiene gripe?*
Have you a cough? With phlegm?	*¿Tiene Tos? ¿Con Flema?*
Sputum/Spit? What color?	*¿Esputo/Escupe? ¿De qué color?*
What color was the phlegm?	*¿Que color tienen las flemas?*
How much? For how long?	*¿Cuánto? ¿Por cuánto tiempo?*
Spit or cough up blood?	*¿Escupe o tose sangre?*
Where have you pain at breathing?	*¿Dónde tiene usted dolor al respirar?*
Have you...?	*¿Tiene...?*
...Shortness Of Breath (SOB)	*...Corto Respiración*
...Shortness Of Breath (SOB)	*...Falta de aire*
...Shortness Of Breath	*...Corto De Resuelo/Respirar*
...Difficult Respiration	*...Respiración Difícil*
...Difficulty Breathing	*...Dificultad al Respirar*
With work or walking?	*¿Con trabajo o caminado?*
Do you have asthma or wheezing?	*¿Tiene asma o silbido?*
Do you have to wake up at night...?	*¿Tiene que despiertar en la noche...?*
...to breath?	*...a respirar?*
How many times?	*¿Cuántas veces?*
How many pillows do you have to use?	*¿Cuántas almohadas tiene (usted) que usar?*
Do you have shortness of breath climbing a few stairs?	*¿Se le corta la respiración cuando subio las escaleras?*
How many stairs?	*¿Cuántas escaleras?*
Any difficulty walking 2-3 blocks?	*¿Algunas dificultades al caminar dos o tres cuadras?*
Do you have to rest to breath?	*¿Tiene usted que descansar para respirar?*

For how long do you rest?	¿Por cuánto tiempo tiene usted que descansar?
Do your ankles swell? (SOA)	¿Se le hinchan los tobillos?
Smoke? How many packs a day?	¿Fuma? ¿Cuántos paquetes al día?
For how many years?	¿Por cuántos años?
Have you ever been treated for...?	¿Ha sido tratado alguna ves por...?
...Pneumonia or pleurisy?	...Pulmonia o Pleuresía?
...TB or Bronchitis?	...Tuberculosis (TB) o Bronquitis?
Have you been given an immunization for TB?	¿Le pusieron vacuna contra la TB?
Have you taken a test for TB?	¿Te tomaron la prueba para TB?
Have you had a test for TB?	¿Le han hecho la prueba para TB?
Was it positive or negative?	¿Fue positiva o negativa?
Have you had taken an x-ray of your chest?	¿Le han tomado radiografia del pecho?
Was it normal or abnormal?	¿Fue normal o anormal?

Cultural Note: It is more courteous to say "Please breathe" than to say "Breathe please." Therefore, "Favor de respirar" is favored over the rather impolite "Respirar, por favor!"

Cultural Note: There are many, many words for a "cold" or having URI symptoms. "Resfrío" is useful to describe the "common cold." "Gripe" (pronounced "grip-ah") is a flu. You can "have" a flu, but you do not "have" a cold, you simply "are with cold." Therefore, you would say "¿Está resfriado o tiene gripe?" (Are you with cold or do you have the flu?) It is possible to have one, the other, or both.

Spanish Note: You may hear two words associated with an M.D., they are "médico" and "doctor." "Médico" refers to a physician while "Doctor" usually refers to a PhD. Although "Médico" is more correct, each may be used when referring to a physician.

Spanish Note: "Escalofríos" is the Spanish word for chills. This may simply mean the patient feels cold and needs a blanket. "Tembladera" (sounds kind of like "tremble-dera") is used to describe the chills which lead to shaking.

CARDIAC: chest pain, palpitations, shortness of breath (SOB), shortness of breath on exertion (SOBOE), PND, orthopnea, SOA (ankle edema), murmur, HTN, past MI

Please refer to "Chest Pain" in the PAIN section for a more complete work-up of chest pain of undetermined origin.

Heart Disease	*Enfermedad Del Corazón*
Heart Failure	*Falla Cardiaca*
Heart Failure	*Falla Del Corazón*
Heart Broken	*Muerto De Pena*
Heart Attack	*Ataque de Corazón*
Heart Murmur	*Soplo Del Corazón*
Heart Burn	*Acedía/Agruras*

Boring (Penetrating)	*Penetrante*
Burning	*Que Quema/Ardiente*
Continuous	*Continuo*
Deep	*Hondo*
Dull	*Sordo*
Heavy	*Pesado*
Intense	*Intensivo*
Intermittent	*Intermitente*
Light/Moderate	*Ligero/Moderado*
Pressure	*Con Presión*
Referred	*Referido*
Ripping	*Rasgante*
Severe	*Severo/Fuerte*
Sharp	*Agudo*
Shooting	*Punzante*
Tearing	*Desgarrante*
That Moves	*Que Se Mueve*
Throbbing (Pulsatile)	*Pulsante*
Tightness	*Tirantez/Estrecho, Ceñido*

Do you have chest pain or angina?	*¿Tiene dolor de pecho o angina de pecho?*
Ever had heart pain (at any time)?	*¿Le duele el corazón (algunes veces)?*
For how long?	*¿Por cuánto tiempo?*
Do you feel sweaty?	*¿Se siente sudado?*
Do you have high blood pressure?	*¿Tiene alta presion (de sangre)?*

Do you have a heart murmur? ("do you have a blow in the heart?")	¿Tiene un soplo en el corazón?
Have you ever had a heart attack?	¿Ha tenido un ataque de corazón?
You wake up during the night…?	¿Se despierta durante la noche…?
…for shortness of breath?	…por corta la respiración?
…for shortness of breath?	…por falta de aire?
How many times?	¿Cuántas veces?
How many pillows do you have to use?	¿Cuántas almohadas tiene usted que usar?
Any difficulty walking 2-3 blocks?	¿Algunas dificultades al caminar dos o tres cuadras?
Do you have to rest to breath?	¿Tiene usted que descansar para respirar?
For how long do you rest?	¿Por cuánto tiempo tiene usted que descansar?
Do you have shortness of breath climbing some stairs? One floor?	¿Se le corto respiración subiendo unas escaleras? ¿Un piso?
How many stairs?	¿Cuántas escaleras?
Smoke? How many packs a day?	¿Fuma? ¿Cuántos paquetes al día?
Do your ankles swell? (SOA)	¿Se le hinchan los tobillos?
Have you had…	¿Se le han…?
…Swelling of the hands, face, legs?	…Inchado las manos, el rostro (la cara), las piernas?
…rapid heart rate?	…pulsaciones rápidas del corazón?
Have you had palpitations?	¿Ha tenido palpitaciones?

C/C/E	= Cyanosis/Claudication/Edema
COR	= Heart
CVA	= Cerebral Vascular Accident (Stroke)
DOE	= Dyspnea on Exersion (same as SOBOE)
HJR	= Hepato-Jugular Reflex
HTN	= Hypertension (High Blood Pressure)
JVD	= Jugular Venous Distention
JVP	= Jugular Venous Pressure
MI	= Myocardial Infarction (Heart Attack)
ORTHOPNEA	= S.O.B. only while laying down
PND	= Paroxysmal Nocturnal Dyspnea
ROM	= Range of Motion
S1/S2	= First and Second Heart Sounds
SOA	= Swelling of the Ankles
SOB	= Shortness of breath
SOBOE	= Shortness of Breath on Exersion

BREASTS pain, discharge, trauma, lumps

Breasts (Men)	*Pecho*
Breasts (Women)	*Senos /Las Pechos*
Discharge	*Desecho/Flujo*
Trauma	*Trauma*
Lumps	*Pelotitas*
Masses "Balls"	*Masas/Bolitas/Bolas*
Armpit	*Axila/Sobaco*
Cancer	*Cáncer*
Benign	*Benigno*
Tumor	*Tumor*

Any pain in your breasts?	*¿Algun dolor en sus pechós/ senos?*
Any discharge from your breasts?	*¿Algun desecho de sus senos?*
...White liquid	*...Liquido blanco*
...Milk	*...Leche*
...Blood	*...Sangre*
Injury to your breasts?	*¿Se ha lastimado los senos?*
Have you had any new lumps or masses in your breasts?	*¿Ha tenido algunas bolas o masas nuevas en sus senos?*
With pain? Hard or soft?	*¿Con dolores? ¿Duros o suave?*
Any masses/lumps in your armpit?	*¿Algunas masas/bolitas/ bolas/ pelotitas en sus axilas?*
Stationary or mobile?	*¿Estacionarios ó mobiles?*
Have you had a mammogram (an x-ray of the breasts)? What date?	*¿Ha tenido una mamografia (una rayos equis del senos)? ¿Qué fecha?*

GENITOURINARY dysuria, frequency, urgency, nocturia,
hesitancy, hematuria, discharges, STDs, sexual function

Bed Pan/Urinal	*El Bacin/El Orinal*
Urinate ("Make Pee")	*Orinar/"Hacer Pipi"*

Do you have pain or burning at *¿Tiene dolor o ardor al orinar?*
urination?

How many times do you uri- *¿Cuántas veces orina cada día?*
nate each day?

Do you have the urge to uri- *¿Tiene le ganas de orinar muy*
nate frequently (often)? *frecuentemente (a menudo)?*

How often do you... urinate? *¿Qué tan seguido... orinar?*

Do you have to wait for the *¿Tiene que esperar para que le*
urine to flow (come out)? *salga la orina?*

Do you have blood in the *¿Tiene usted sangre en la orina?*
urine?

The urine... *La orina...*

...bloody *...con sangre (with blood)?*

...cloudy *...turbia?*

...is it normal *...está normal?*

Urinate during the night? *¿Orinas durante la noche?*

You wake up during the *¿Se despierta durante la noche...?*
night...? To urinate? *¿A orinar?*

How many times in the night? *¿Cuántas veces en la noche?*

Do you have frequent infec- *¿Tiene infección con frecuencía?*
tions? (Frequently?) *(¿Frecuentemente?)*

Do you have kidney stones *¿Tiene cálculos en el riñón (mal de*
(stone disease)? *piedra)?*

Do you have loss of urine? *¿Tiene pérdida de orina?*

Any abnormal discharge *¿Algunas desechos (secreciones)*
(secretions)? *anormales?*

Have you had venereal *¿Has tenido enfermedad venéreas?*
disease?

Do you have problems with *¿Tiene problems con relaciones*
sex? *(sexuales)?*

Do you have sex frequently? *¿Tiene relaciones (sexuales) con*
frecuencia?

Cultural Note: "Cálculo en el riñón," literally, "Stone in the kidney" is a correct medical phrase but it will only bewilder most of
your hispanic patients. "Stone Sickness," or "Mal de piedra" is a
time honored colloquialism to describe kidney stones.

GASTROINTESTINAL weight changes, pain, appetite (changes), nausea/vomiting, diarrhea, constipation, melena, hematochezia, hematemesis, hemorrhoids, clay colored stools, jaundice/hepatitis, gall bladder disease, excessive gas, burping, or flatus

---

Diarrhea/Constipation	Diarrea/Estreñimiento
Nausea/Violent Nausea	Náusea/Basca
Stool	Deposiciones/"Pupu"
Stool	Excremento/"Caca"
Stool	Las Heces
Bed Pan	La "Chata"/El Bacin
To Vomit/Vomit	Vomitar/Vómito
Defecate "Make Stool"	Defecar/"Hacer Caca"
To Move The Bowels	Obrar

How much do you weigh?	¿Cuánto pesa?
Your normal weight?	¿Su peso normal?
What is your normal weight?	¿Cual es su peso normal?
Changes recently… in your weight?	¿Cambios recientemente… en su peso?
How much weight have you gained/lost?	¿Cuánto peso ha subido/bajado?
How many pounds?	¿Cuántas libras?
How is your appetite?	¿Cómo está su apetito?
Your digestion, good?	¿La digestión - buena?
Problems with digestion?	¿Problemas con la digestión?
Do you have nausea or vomiting?	¿Tiene náusea o vómito?
Do you have the urge to vomit?	¿Tiene usted ganas de vomitar?
Vomit of what kind?	¿Vómitos de qué clase?
Describe the vomit.	Describa el vomito.
You feel that you have vomiting after eating?	¿Siente que tiene que vomitar después de comer?
Do you have to vomit while eating?	¿Tiene que vomitar al comer?
Do you have to vomit after eating?	¿Tiene que vomitar después de comer?
How much time (in minutes) after eating?	¿Cuantos tiempo (en minutos) depués de comer?

Do you have vomit with blood?	*¿Tiene vómito con sangre?*
Vomited blood at any time?	*¿Vomita sangre a veces?*
The color of coffee?	*¿Color de café?*
Cough up blood?	*¿Tuese sangre?, ¿Tose sangre?*
Do you have diarrhea or constipation?	*¿Tiene diarrea o estreñimiento?*
Do you have cramps or colic?	*¿Tiene calambres o cólicos?*
Do you have hemorrhoids?	*¿Tiene almorranas (hemorroides)?*
Do you have blood in the stool?	*¿Tiene sangre en los deposiciones (en las haces)?*
Any stools the color of clay (with the color of clay)?	*¿Algunos deposiciones la color de barro (son de color de barro)?*
Any stools the color of black?	*¿Algunos deposiciones de color negro?*
When did you last have a bowel movement?	*¿Cuándo obró por última vez?*
Of what color?	*¿De qué color?*
Have you had "yellow skin" (jaundice)?	*¿Has tenido piel amarilla?*
Have you had hepatitis?	*¿Has tenido hepatitis?*
Have you had gall bladder attacks?	*¿Has tenido ataque de la vesícular biliar?*
Have you had gall stones?	*¿Has tenido cálculo biliar/ piedras biliar?*
Do you feel food is stuck in your throat?	*¿Se siente alimento atorado en la garganta?*
Use laxatives?	*¿Usas laxativos?*
Do you have a lot of gas?	*¿Tiene mucho gas?*
Do you have a lot of burping?	*¿Tiene eructa mucho?*
Pass a lot of gas (farts)?	*¿Pasa muchos gas (pedos)?*

Cultural Note: "Urine" is a common word in Spanish, however, "stool" is not. "Deposiciones" was chosen by consensus of Latin-American M.D.s working in the Los Angeles area as being a reasonable substitute. "Excremento" may also be useful for stool though tends to be above the vocabulary level of many. "Las Heces" seems to work well in the western states. "Pupú" or "Caca" are child expressions for stool and can be used in a pinch, although I would advice against using them with adults. "Pedo" is common Mexican slang for "fart."

HEMATOLOGICAL history of anemia (specify), easy bruising,
persisting bleeding, HIV antibody test

Have you had anemia (at times/at any time)?	¿Has tenido anemia (a veces/ alguna vez)?
Do you have loss of blood?	¿Tiene pérdida de sangre?
Blood from where?	¿Sangre de dónde?
How much blood?	¿Cuánta sangre?
What medicines have you been taking?	¿Qué medicinas ha estado tomando?
Iron, vitamins, other medicines?	¿Hierro, vitaminas, otra medicinas?
Have you had a transfusion of blood?	¿Ha tenido una tranfusion (infusion) de sangre?
Bleed easily?	¿Sangra facíl/facílmente?
Do you have any bleeding tendency?	¿Tiene alguna tendencia a sangrar?
Do you have hemophilia?	¿Tiene hemofilia?
Do you have nose bleeds?	¿Tiene usted sangrado de nariz?
Does your nose bleed?	¿Le sangra la nariz?
Do you have cuts which are slow healing?	¿Tiene cortadas que se curan lentamente?
Has anyone in your family have…	¿Hay alguien en su familia que haya tenido…
…Problems with anesthesia?	…Problemas con anestesia?
…Bleeding tendency?	…Tendencia a sangrar?
…Hemophilia?	…Hemofilia?
…Nose bleeds?	…Sangrado por la nariz?
…Phlebitis?	…Flebitis?
Do you bruise easily?	¿Fácilmente se moretea?
Do you bleed easily?	¿Sangra fácilmente?
Does it take a long time for your blood to clot?	¿Dura mucho tiempo para que su sangre se coágular?
Have you ever had a tested for AIDS?	¿Le han hecho una prueba de SIDA?
Was it positive or negative?	¿Fue positivo o negativo?

ENDOCRINE thyroid problems (hot/cold intolerance), easy
fatiguability, hx of polyuria/polydipsia, diabetes, neck swelling,
other.

Do you have thyroid problems?   *¿Tiene problemas con la tiroides?*

Do you have enlarged or inflamed glands?   *¿Tiene glándulas crecidas o inflamadas?*

Do you feel hot or cold all of the time?   *¿Siente frío o calor todo el tiempo?*

Does hot bother you (more than before)?   *¿Le molesta el calor (más qué antes)?*

Does cold bother you (more than before)?   *¿Le molesta el frío (más qué antes)?*

Do you tire easily?   *¿Se cánsá facil?*

Do you have thirst all the time?   *¿Tiene sed todo el tiempo?*

How many times do you drink liquids each day?   *¿Cuántas veces toma liquidos cada día?*

How many times do you urinate each day?   *¿Cuántas veces orina cada día?*

Do you have high blood sugar?   *¿Tiene alta azúcar en la sangre?*

Do you have diabetes?   *¿Tiene diabetes?*

You use insulin or a diet to control your diabetes?   *¿Usa insulina o una dieta para controlar su diabetes?*

How much insulin in the morning? NPH/Regular? In the afternoon?   *¿Cuántas insulina en la mañana? ¿NPH (Ene-Pe-Hache)/Regular? ¿En la tarde?*

Have you been losing your hair?   *¿Ha pérdido su pelo?*

Have you seen changes in your skin or hair recently?   *¿A visto cambios en su piel o pelo recientemente?*

Any falling out of hair recently?   *¿Alguna caida del cabello recientemente?*

Any changes in the size of your glove or hat?   *¿Algunes cambios en la medida de sus guantes o sombrero?*

MUSCULOSKELETAL joint pains, redness, swelling, decreased function, myalgia, back pain, other.

Joints	Articulación/Coyuntura	Knee bone	Hueso de la Rodilla
Muscles	Músculos	Legs	Piernas
Back	Espalda	Knee	Rodillas
Bones	Huesos	Calves	Pantorrillas
Arms	Brazos	Feet	Pies
Shoulder	Hombro	Ankle	Tobillos
Clavicle	Clavícula	Toes	Dedos del pie
Elbow	Codo	Heel	Talón
Forearm	Antebrazo	Sole	Planta del pie
Hands	Manos		
Fingers	Dedos	Sprain	Torcedura
Thumb	Pulgar	Bowlegged	Corvo
Wrists	Muñecas	Fracture	Fractura

Have you had any joints swollen or red?	¿Ha tenido algunas coyunturas hinchadas o rojas?
Is it difficult to use your hands/feet?	¿Es difícil usar sus manos o pies?
Any muscle pain?	¿Algun dolor múscular?
Do you have any problems with your joints?	¿Tiene algun problema con sus coyunturas?
Point to where the pain is…	Apunte dónde le duele…
Point with the finger…	Señalar con el dedo…
Do you have arthritis or pain in the joints?	¿Tiene arthritis o dolores en las coyunturas?
Do you have back pain?	¿Tiene dolor de espalda?
Do you have pain which goes from the back to the legs?	¿Tiene dolor que camina de la espalda a las perinas?
Have you noted changes in your (fingers)/(toes)?	¿Ha notado cambios en sus (dedos de la mano)/(dedos de los pies)?
Change in color? Blue? Purple? Black?	¿Cambios de color? ¿Azul? ¿Morado (amoratado)? ¿Negro?
Have you noted coldness en your (fingers)/(toes)?	¿Ha notado frío en sus (dedos de la mano)/(dedos de los pies)?
Swelling?	¿Hinchazón?

MENSTRUAL (BRIEF) menarche, menstrual triad (cycle, duration, dysmenorrhea) vaginal discharge (color, amount, odor, consistency, pain, itching), number of pregnancies, number of deliveries, number of abortions, number of living

(Please see OB/GYN for a more thorough Menstrual History)

At what age did the periods begin?	*¿A qué edad tuvo su primer regla?*
What age did you start to mensturate?	*¿A qué edad empezo su regla/menstraccion?*
When did you have your last period?	*¿Cuándo fue su ultima regla?*
For how many days duration?	*¿Por cuántos días dura?*
How many days do you bleed?	*¿Por cuántos días sangra?*
How many days between your periods?	*¿Cuánto diás entre sus reglas?*
Did you have a normal period?	*¿Tuvo una regla normal?*
Do you have pains with your menses?	*¿Tiene dolor con sus reglas?*
Any unusual bleeding between periods?	*¿Algun sangrado inusual entre reglas/periodos?*
Do you have vaginal discharge/secretions?	*¿Tiene flujós/desechos vaginales?*
Thick or not thick?	*¿Espeso o no espeso?*
A lot of itching? Pain?	*¿Mucho comezón? ¿Dolor?*
How many total pregnancies?	*¿Cuántos embarazos en total?*
How many children have you?	*¿Cuántos niños tiene usted?*
How many children living?	*¿Cuántos niños vivos?*
How many children dead?	*¿Cuántos niños muertos?*
How many miscarriages?	*¿Cuántos malpartos?*
The weight of the last baby?	*¿El peso del último bebé/niño?*
The last delivery...	*¿El último parto...?*
...Short or Long?	*...Corto o Largo?*
...Have any problems?	*...Tuvo algunos problemas?*
When was your last Pap test?	*¿Cuándo fue su ultima prueba de /Pap (Papanicolado)?*

SKIN rashes, chronic problems, tattoos, scars, others

Have you had any difficulties with your skin?	*¿Ha tenido dificultad alguna con su piel?*
Do you have or have you had at any time...?	*¿Tiene o ha tenido alguna vez...?*

...Chronic problems (with your skin)	*...Problemas Cronicos (con su piel)*
...Skin diseases	*...Enfermedad de la piel*
...Rashes	*...Salpullidos/ronchas/ erupciónes*
...Scars	*...Cicatrizes*
...Tattoos	*...Tatuajes*
...Bleeding Tendency	*...Tendencia a sangrar*
...Bruise	*...Moretón/Contusión*
...Bump/Lump	*...Bulto/Protuberancia*
...Burn	*...Quemadura*
...Cut	*...Cortada/Cortadura*
...Dermatitis	*...Dermatitis*
...Gash	*...Cuchillada*
...Herpes	*...Herpes*
...Hives (Urticaria)	*...Urticaria/Ronchas*
...Itch	*...Comezón/Picazón*
...Jaundice ("Yellow Skin")	*...Piel Amarilla/Ictericia*
...Lice	*...Piojos*
...Mites	*...Ácaros*
...Mole	*...Lunar*
...Pimple	*...Grano/Barro*
...Ringworm (Tinea)	*...Tiña/Tinea*
...Skin-Cracked	*...Grieta*
...Skin-Discolored	*...Paños*
...Skin-Dry	*...Piel Seca*
...Skin-Irritaion	*...Irritación de la piel*
...Skin-Oily	*...Piel Grasosa*
...Sunburn	*...Quemadura de sol*
...Wart	*...Verruga*
...Wound	*...Herida*

NEUROPSYCHIATRIC dizziness, vertigo, syncope, seizures, parasthesias, tremors, changes in memory, speech problems, emotional problems (depression, suicide, anxiety, history of past psychological care)

Do you have or have you had at any time...	*¿Tiene o ha tenido alguna vez...?*
...**Dizziness**	*...Mareos*
...**Vertigo**	*...Vértigo*
...**Fainting Spell**	*...Desmayo/Sincope*
...**Convulsions**	*...Convulsiones/Ataques*
...**Epilepsy**	*...Epilepsia*
...**Tremors**	*...Temblores*
...**Paralysis**	*...Parálisis*
...**Unusual/Weird Sensations On Your Skin**	*...Sensaciones Inusuales/Raras En Su Piel*
...**Changes In Memory**	*...Cambios De Memoria*
...**Loss Of Conciousness**	*...Pérdida Del Conocimiento*
...**Loss Of Memory**	*...Pérdida Del Memoria*
...**Loss Of Recall**	*...Pérdida Del Recuerdo*
...**Problems When Talking**	*...Problemas al Hablar*
...**Emotional Problems**	*...Problemas Emocionales*
...**Anxiety**	*...Anxiedad/Ansiedad/Ansia*
...**Depression**	*...Depresión*
...**Suicide**	*...Suicidio*
When? What date?	*¿Cuándo? ¿Qué fecha?*
For how long?	*¿Por cuánto tiempo?*
Have you ever been treated by a Psychiatrist or Psycologist?	*¿Ha sido tratado por un psiquiatria o psicólogo?*
Have you ever been treated in a psychiatric hospital?	*¿Ha sido tratado en una hospital psiquiatrico?*
Have you had mental problems in the past?	*¿Ha tenido problemas mentales en el pasado?*
Have you had a history of mental problems?	*¿Ha tenido historia de problemas mentales?*
Do you know...?	*¿Sabe usted...?*
...**What's Your Name**	*...Como se llama*
...**Where You Are**	*...Dónde Esta*
...**What Day It Is**	*...Qué Dia Es*

SEXUAL HISTORY

Do you have or have you had (at any time)...?	*¿Tiene o ha tenido (alguna vez)...?*
...Candidiasis	*...Moniliasis*
...Canker Sores	*...Postemilla*
...Chancre	*...Chancro*
...Chlamydia	*...Clamidia*
...Condyloma	*...Condiloma*
...Gonorrhea	*...Gonorrea*
...Herpes (Genital)	*...Herpes Genital*
...Oral Lesions	*...Fuegos En La Boca*
...Syphilis	*...Sífilis*
...Trichomonas	*...Tricomonas*
...Warts (Genital)	*...Verruga Genital*
Do you use contraception?	*¿Usa usted contraceptivos?*
What kind of birth control have you been using...?	*¿Qué clase de control de nacimiento ha usado...?*
"How do you take care of yourself?" (slang for contraception)	*"Como se cuida"*
...Condoms	*...Condónes*
...Contraceptive Foam	*...Espuma Anticonceptivas*
...Contraceptive Pills	*...Pastillas Anticonceptivas*
...IUD (intrauterine device)	*...El Aparato/Dispositivo Intrauterino (DIU)*
...Diaphragm	*...Diafragma*
Had you any problems (with the pills)?	*¿Tiene problemas (con las pastillas)?*
What age did you start having sex?	*¿A qué edad comenzó usted a tener relaciónes (sexuales)?*
Are you sexually active?	*¿Esta sexualmente activo?*
How many times a week have you sex with your spouse?	*¿Cuántos veces a la semana a tenido relaciónes (sexuales) con su esposa?*
Any problems having or enjoying sex?	*¿Algun problema al tener o gozar el sexo?*
Is your sexual functioning affected by your present illness?	*¿Es su funcionamiento sexual afectado por presente enfermedad?*

Do you have more than one sexual partner?	¿Tiene más que un compañero (sexual)?
How many total different partners have you had?	¿Cuántos diferentes compañeros tiene usted?
Have you ever had a venereal disease?	¿Ha tenido enfermedad venerea?
Do you have any penile/ vaginal discharge?	¿Tiene algun flujó del pene/ vaginal?
Do you have sex with men, women or both?	¿Tuvo sexo con un hombre, una mujer o ambos?
Do you have sex with different men or women?	¿Tuvo relaciónes (sexuales) con diferentes hombres o mujeres?

MEN

Problems having or maintaining an erection?	¿Problemas teniendo o manteniendo erección?
Problems ejaculating/ orgasm/ "coming?"	¿Problemas al eyacular/ orgasmo/o "al venirse?"
Too slow?	¿Demasiado lento?
Not soon enough?	¿No tan pronto?

WOMEN

Do you have pain during...?	¿Tiene usted dolor durante ...?
...Sexual Intercourse?	...Relaciónes (sexuales)?
...the Penetration?	...La penetración?
Do you have difficulty having orgasm?	¿Tiene dificultades teniendo orgasmo?

BOTH

Is this a major problem?	¿Es este un problema grande?
For how long?	¿Por cuánto tiempo?
Have you had any help before?	¿Ha tenido alguna ayuda anteriormente?
Would you like help?	¿Le gustaria tener ayuda?

Cultural Note: Hispanic women tend to be very shy and will not freely discuss their sex life. Often times simply mentioning the word "sexuales" is sufficiently uncomfortable for the patient to elicit a series of "no" responses to all matters sexual. Therefore, the correct medical phrase for sexual intercourse, "relaciónes sexuales," is shortened to simply "relaciónes" (the "sexuales" is put in brackets for completeness sake, you don't have to actually say the word). The patient should understand from context what "relations" means..

HIV SYMPTOMS

Any reason for which to suspect you have AIDS?	¿Alguna razón por la cual usted sospecha tener SIDA?
Have you ever had a tested for AIDS?	¿Le han hecho una prueba de SIDA?
Was it positive or negative?	¿Fue positivo o negativo?
Do you use IV drugs or share syringes/needles with other people?	¿Usa drogas intravenosas o compartido jeringas/agujas con otras personas?
Have you received a blood transfusion in the past ten years?	¿Ha recibido tranfusion de sangre en los pasedos 10 (diez) años?
Mother with AIDS?	¿Madre con SIDA?
Your mother had AIDS?	¿Su madre tuvo SIDA?
Visit prostitutes?	¿Visita prostitutas?
Oral Sex/Rectal Sex?	¿Sexo oral/Sexo por el ano?
Do you have or have you had (at any time)…?	¿Tiene o ha tenido (alguna vez)…?
…Fatigue/Weakness	…Fatiga/Debilidad
…Weight loss	…Pérdido peso
…Diarrhea	…Diarrea
…Cough/colds with frequency (Often)	…Tosa o resfriós con frecuencia
…Pneumonia	…Pulmonia
…Swelling or tender glands (or hard nodes) in the neck	…Inflamaciones o tiernos glandulas (o nudos duros) en el cuello
…Night Sweats	…Sudores En La Noche
…Skin changes (dark spots)	…Cambios en la piel (manchas oscuras)

THE PHYSICAL EXAM

- GENERAL COMMANDS
- VITAL SIGNS
- HEAD/EARS/EYES/NOSE/THROAT
- NEUROMUSCULAR
- POSITIONING OF THE PATIENT

GENERAL COMMANDS

Tell me.../Let me...	*Dígame.../Déjeme...*
Stand up "On foot"...	*Póngase de pie...*
Stand up here	*Párese aquí*
Sit down...	*Siéntese...*
On the bed, on your back, please!	*¡En la cama, boca arriba, por favor!*
Turn Over "To the reverse"	*¡Voltéese! ¡A la vuelta!*
Breath with the mouth...	*Respire con su boca...*
Hold your breath...	*Mantenga su respiración...*
Follow...the light...	*Siga...la luz...*
Look At...my finger...	*Mire...mi dedo...*
Pain when I push?	*Duele cuando le empujó?*
Can you show me with one finger?	*¿Puede enseñarme con un dedo?*
Point to where the pain is...	*Apunte dónde le duele...*
Point with the finger...	*Señalar con el dedo...*
I need to have a sample of blood/urine.	*Necesito una muestra de su sangre/orina.*
I am going to take your...	*Le voy a tomar su(s)...*
...Blood Pressure	*...Presion De Sange*
...Pulse	*...Pulso*
...Temperature	*...Temperatura*
I am going to listen to your...	*Le voy a escuchar a su(s)...*
...Heart	*...Corazón*
...Lungs	*...Pulmones*
...Abdomen	*...Abdomen*
Make a fist	*Haga un puño*
Hold your breath	*Mantenga la respiration*
Do like this (mimic)...	*Haga así...*

VITAL SIGNS

Come with me...	*Venga con migo...*
Stand up "On foot"...	*Póngase de pie...*
Up on the scale...	*Súbase a la báscula...*
Take a step down...	*Tome un paso abajo...*
How tall are you (in feet)?	*¿Cuánto mide usted (en pies)?*
Sit down...	*Siéntese...*
Lift up your sleeve...	*Súbase la manga...*
Give me your hand...	*Deme la mano...*
Let me take your pulse...	*Déjeme tomarle el pulso...*
I am going to take your...	*Le voy a tomar su...*
...Blood Pressure	*...Presion De Sange*
...Pulse	*...Pulso*
...Temperature	*...Temperatura*
Open/Close the mouth...	*Abra/Cierre la boca...*
Under the tongue...	*Debajo de le lengua...*
I am going to listen to your...	*Le voy a escuchar a su...*
...Heart	*...Corazón*
...Lungs	*...Pulmones*
Breath deeply (by mouth)...	*Respire profundo (por la boca)...*
Again ("another time")...	*Otra vez...*
Cough...	*Tosa...*
Please go to room/door number (__).	*Favor de pasar al cuarto/ puerta numero (__).*

Undress, please...	*Desvístase, por favor...*
Remove the clothes...	*Quítese la ropa...*
From the waist up/down...	*De la cintura arriba/abajo...*
Remove your panties...	*Quitese las pantaletas (calzones)...*
Remove everything...	*Quitese todo...*
Put on this (gown)...	*Póngase esto (camisón)...*
Put on the clothes...	*Póngase la ropa...*
You can get dressed.	*Usted se puede vestir.*

I need to have a sample of your ...urine./...blood	*Necesito una muestra de su ...orina./...sangre*
The doctor will be in later.	*El doctor vendra más tarde.*
The doctor is going to examine you.	*El doctor va a examinarla.*

HEENT-Head, Ears, Eyes, Nose, Throat (BRIEF)

HEENT: HEAD: signs of trauma, masses, tenderness, scalp, bruit EARS: gross hearing, external, pinna, canal, TM, landmarks, mobility, light reflex, Weber, Renne EYES: acuity, visual fields, EOM, conjunctivae, sclera, limbus, corneal reflex, PERRL, disc, cup, artery, vein, A/V ratio NOSE: patency, septum intact, mucosa (signs of inflammation), discharge SINUSES: palp for tenderness, frontal, mastoid, maxillary, transillumination (prn) MOUTH: inspection of lips, tongue, mucosa, teeth, THROAT: pharynx, tonsils, uvular deviation, gag reflex NECK: supple, ROM, thyroid exam, trachea position, carotid pulse, bruits, lymph node palpation, JVD

Examine the head for trauma.

Examine the eyes for PERRL/EOMI/RETINA

Open/Close the eyes...	*Abra/Cierre los ojos...*
Follow the light...	*Siga la luz...*
Follow my finger with the eyes	*Siga me dedo con los ojos*
Look at the light...	*Mira la luz...*
Look at a spot on the ceiling...	*Mira a una mancha en el cielo...*
And don't move your eyes...	*Y no mueve sus ojos...*
Look up/down...	*Mira arriba/abajo...*
Read this line	*Lea esta linea*
What color do you see?	*¿Qué color ve usted?*
Look me in the nose & tell me when you see my finger...	*Véame a la nariz y dígame cuando vea mi dedo*

Examine the Ears & Neck Mobility:

Move your head right/left...	*Mueve su cabeza al la derecha/ izquierda...*
Don't move your head...	*No mueve su cabeza...*
Move your head...	*Mueva su cabeza...*
...to the right	*...a la derecha*
...to the left	*...a la izquierda*
...forward	*...al frente*
...and to the back	*...y para atrás*
Have pain in the ear? (pull on pinna)	*¿Tiene dolor en el oído?*

In which ear do you hear the buzzing [from tuning fork] the most?	*¿En cuál oreja oye el zumbido mejor?*

Examine the nose with otoscope:

Examine the Mouth:

Open/Close the mouth...	*Abra/Cierre la boca...*
Stick out the tongue...	*Saque la lengua...*
Say, Ah!!	*¡Diga, "Ah!!"*
Lift your tongue.	*Levante la lengua...*
I'm sorry (after gag tested)...	*Lo siento...*
Move your tongue right/left...	*Mueve su lengua a la derecha/ izquierda...*

Examine the Neck

Let me move your neck...	*Déjeme mover su cuello...*
Swallow...Pass Saliva...	*Trague...Pasa saliva...*
Breath with the mouth...	*Respire con su boca...*
Hold your breath...	*Mantenga su respiración...*

Examine Sinuses by Tapping:

Pain?	*¿Dolor?*

CRANIAL NERVES

- I   Smell (primary scents) or by patient report
- II   Vision (direct/ concentual reflexes)
- III EOM (all EOM except...)
- IV   EOM (sup. oblique - inferior/lateral gaze)
- VI   EOM (abducens - abduction)
- V   Sensory (facial: V1-ophthalmic, V2-maxillary, V3-mandibular) if abnormal, test hot/cold, light touch, and corneal. Motor (masseter, temporal)
- VII Facial expression, platysmus, raise eyebrow, frown, smile, close eyes tight, show upper, lower teeth, puff out cheeks
- VIII Hearing, whisper, Webber and if indicated, Renne
- IX/X Gag reflex, midline uvula
- XI   Trapezius and sternocleidomastoid
- XII Protrude tongue midline

Let's see! Let's see!	*¡A ver, a ver!*
Let's see where!	*¡A ver dónde!*

NEUROMUSCULAR EXAM

Tell me.../Let me...	*Dígame.../Déjeme...*
This is an exam of your...	*Este es un examen de su...*
...Muscles	*...Músculos*
... Feelings	*...Sensaciónes*
...Nerves	*...Nervios*
...Strength	*...Fuerza*
...Balance	*... Equilibrio*
Try to move your...	*Trate de mover...*
...Arms	*...Los brazos*
...Legs	*...Los piernas*
Make a fist	*Haga un puño*
Repeat the words...I'm going to say	*Repita las palabras...que voy a decir*
Squeeze my fingers in your hand. Harder.	*Apriete mis dedos en su mano. Más duro.*

Do like this with your ...	*Haga así con su(s)...*

Open/Close your eyes...	*Abra/Cierre los ojos...*
Relax and let me move your...	*Relájese y déjeme mover su(s)...*
...Fingers/Toes	*...Dedos/Dedos del pies*
...Arms/Legs	*...Brazos/Piernas*
...Hands/Feet	*...Manos/Pies*
Do you feel me when I touch?	*¿Me siente cuando lo toco?*
Tell me if this is...	*Dígame si esto es...*
...Sharp Or Not Sharp	*...Agudo O No Agudo*
...Hot Or Cold	*...Caliente O Frío*
...Up Or Down	*...Hacia Arriba O Hacia Abajo*
...Toward Me Or Toward You	*...Hacia Mí O Hacia Usted*
...Vibration or No Vibration	*...Vibración o No Vibración*
Don't let me move you...	*No me deje moverlo...*
Don't move please...	*No se mueva por favor...*
Stand up "Put on foot"...	*Póngase de pie...*

Cultural Note: Although a common contrast in English, "dull" is not a common contrast to "sharp" in Spanish. Don't use "dull" (sordo) in contrast to "sharp" (agudo) because your patients will stare at you in bewilderment. I have found "agudo" (sharp) and "no agudo" (not sharp) as good contrasts. "Punta" (point) and "Sin punta" (without point) can also be used.

POSITIONING PHRASES

Sit Up	*Siéntese*
Lie Down - Face Up	*Acuéstese-Boca Arriba*
Lie Down - Face Down	*Acuéstese-Boca Abajo*
Lift Yourself	*Levántese*
Up On The Table	*Súbase A La Mesa*
Get On...The Stomach	*Póngase De Estómago*
Get On...Hands & Knees	*Póngase En Manos Y Rodillas*
Bend Your...Knees/Arms	*Doble Su...Rodillas/Brazo*
Right Side/Left Side	*Lado Derecha/Lado Izquierda*
On the other side (Turn Over)	*A La Vuelta*
Raise The Arms/Legs	*Levante Los Brazos/Piernas*
Right/Left	*Derecha/Izquierda*
Wait Here	*Espere Aquí*

POSITIONING COMMANDS

Bend	*Doble*	Point	*Apunte*
Blow	*Sople*	Push/Pull	*Empuje/Tire*
Breath	*Respire*	Put On...	*Póngase...*
Call	*Llame*	Put/Place	*Ponga*
Chew	*Mastique*	Relax/Rest	*Relájese/Descanse*
Close/Open	*Cierre/Abra*	Remove	*Quite*
Drink	*Tome/Beba*	Repeat	*Repita/ Otra Vez*
Eat	*Coma*	Return	*Regrese*
Exhale	*Exhale*	Say "Ah!"	*Dígame "¡Ah!"*
Extend	*Extienda*	Sign	*Firme*
Fast/Slow	*Rapido/ Despacio*	Sit Down	*Siéntese*
Follow	*Siga*	Squeeze	*Apriete*
Give Me	*Déme*	Stay	*Quédese*
Go	*Vaya*	Step	*Tome Paso*
Grab/Hold	*Agarre*	Stop	*Deje, Alta*
Hard/Easy	*Fuerte/Suave*	Swallow	*Trague*
Hold (Maintain)	*Mantenga/ Sustenga*	Take (Ingest)	*Tome*
In/Out	*Adentro/ Afuera*	Tell Me	*Dígame*
Inhale	*Inhale*	Touch	*Toque*
Lie Down	*Acquéstese*	Turn (Wind)	*Vire*
Lift	*Levante*	Turn Over	*Voltéese*
Look At...	*Mira*	Turn Over	*A La Vuelta*
Make	*Haga/Hacer*	Up/Down	*Arriba/Abajo*
Move	*Mueva*	Wash	*Lave*
Open/Close	*Abra/Cierre*	Watch/Look	*Mire*

PAIN QUESTIONS

- ## PQRST OF PAIN
  - ### PROVOCATIVE & PALLIATIVE
  - ### QUANTITY & QUALITY
  - ### RADIATION & LOCATION
  - ### SEVERITY & DEBILITY
  - ### TIME OF DAY & DURATION
- ## CHEST PAIN
- ## HEADACHE

- "PQRST" is an easy to remember system for describing any symptom or patient complaint. It provides a fairly detailed analysis of the patients perception of their problem and is quite useful in diagnosis. General PQRST questions are provided in this section.

- *Chest Pain* is briefly described using the PQRST format. This is helpful to determine the origin of chest pain. It's primary focus is on differentiating Cardiac from Non-Cardiac pain.

- *Headache* can be precipitated by no less than 180 known causes. Thankfully, it's generally not necessary to determine the exact origin of a headache in order to render proper treatment. The PQRST questions provide a helpful method to determine which class of headache the patient is suffering (e.g. migraine, cluster, muscle tension).

PQRST of PAIN: Provocative (causative) & Palliative (relieves), Quality & Quantity, Radiation & Location, Severity & Debility, Time associations & Duration.

| Do you have pain? Where? | *¿Tiene dolor? ¿Dónde?* |

PROVOCATIVE/PALLIATIVE

What makes it worse?	*¿Qué lo hace peor?*
What makes it better?	*¿Qué lo hace mejor?*
Is there a position which alleviates the pain?	*¿Hay una posición que alivia el dolor?*
It is worse when...	*¿Está peor cuándo...*
...use the arms/legs	*...usa el brazo/la pierna?*
...walking/at work	*...camina/esta en el trabajo?*
...before/after you eat	*...antes/después de comer?*
It is better when...	*¿Es mejor cuándo*
...you're in bed	*...está en la cama?*
...you're resting	*...está descansando?*

QUALITY/QUANTITY

What kind of pain (do you have)?	*¿Qué clase de dolor (tiene)?*
Sharp/burning?	*¿Agudo/que quema?*
Do you have others problems beginning?	*¿Tuvo otros problemas empezando (este problems)?*
Is this the first time you've had this?	*¿Es la primera vez que ha tenido este?*
Have you had this problem before?	*¿Ha tenido este problema antes?*
Has it been always like this?	*¿Ha sido siempre así?*
Has it been the same as before?	*¿Ha sido egual que antes?*
Began slowly or rapidly?	*¿Empezó despacio o rápido?*
Is it better now or worse or the same?	*¿Está mejor ahora, o peor, o es equal/mismo?*

RADIATION/LOCATION

Where do you feel (the pain)?	*¿Dónde siente (el dolor)?*
Where is the pain?	*¿Dónde está el dolor?*
Can you show me with one finger?	*¿Puede enseñarme con un dedo?*

Point to where the pain is.	*Apunte dónde le duele.*
Where does it run (the pain, the feeling)?	*¿Dónde corre (el dolor, la sensación)?*
...Arm, Back, Jaw, Shoulder	*...Brazo, Espalda, Quijada, Hombros*
Pain that moves? (Radiation)	*¿Dolor que se mueve?*
Feel pain in other parts?	*¿Siente el dolor en otra partes?*
In what other parts?	*¿En qué otras partes?*
Do you have pain here?	*¿Tiene dolor aquí?*

SEVERITY/DEBILITY

Do you have severe pains?	*¿Tiene dolores fuertes?*
How strong is the pain?	*¿Qué tan fuertes es el dolor?*
...light/moderate/severe (strong)?	*...ligero/moderado/severo (fuertes)?*
The pain - wakes you up at night?	*El dolor - ¿le despierta en la noche?*
How many times?	*¿Cuántas veces?*
Can you... work, eat, walk, sleep, have sexual relations?	*¿Puede... trabajar, comer, caminar, dormir, tener relaciónes (sexual)?*
In numbers from 1 to 10, (10 feels strong and 1 feels less), what number is your pain?	*¿En numeros de un a diez (diez siendo fuerte y uno siendo menos), Qué numero es su dolor?*
On a 1 to 10 scale, what number is your pain (10 is the worst, 1 is the least)?	*¿En una escala de uno a diez, Qué numero es su dolor (diez es el peor, una es el menor)?*
On a scale of 1 to 10 (1 being is a little pain and 10 is the worst) how much pain have you now?	*¿En una escale de uno a diez (uno es poco dolor y diez es el peor) cuánto dolor tiene ahora?*

TIME ASSOCIATIONS/DURATION

How long have you had (this problem)?	*¿Cuánto tiempo ha tenido (este problema)?*
When did the pains begin?	*¿Cuándo empezaron los dolores?*
"It Makes" how much time? Minutes/Hours?	*¿Hace cuánto tiempo? ¿Minutos/horas?*
For how long? (Duration)	*¿Por cuánto tiempo?*
When? What date?	*¿Cuándo? ¿Qué fecha?*
When have you more pain?	*¿Cuándo tiene más dolor?*

When have you less pain?	¿Cuándo tiene menos dolor?
...in the Morning	...En la mañana
...Noon "middle day"	...Medio Dias
...the Afternoon	...La Tarde
...at Night	...de Noche
For how long have you each pain?	¿Por cuánto tiempo tiene cada dolor?
How much time between the pains?	¿Cuánto tiempo entre los dolores?

OTHER HIGH UTILITY QUESTIONS

Take medicines for the pain?	¿Toma medicina por el dolor?
The medicines helps?	¿La medicina ayuda?
What are the names of your medicines?	¿Cuál es los nombres du sus medicinas?
Do you have your medicines with you?	¿Tiene sus medicinas con usted?
What have you done for this problem?	¿Qué ha hecho por este problema?
Have you had tests of blood/urine, x-rays, other exams (for this problem)?	¿Ha tendio análisis de la sangre/orina, radiografiás, o ostros exámes (por este problema)?
What were the results? Normal, high, positive?	¿Qué fue el resultado? Normal, alto, positivo?

Spanish Note: "Haga así" ("Do like this...") has great utility and can be used to have the patient mimic your actions. This is an excellent phrase for neuromuscular testing (e.g. Rhomberg, pronator drift, standing on one foot).

Medical Spanish Note: Although much emphasis is given to training in physical diagnosis, remarkably little Spanish is necessary to conduct a complete physical exam. Therefore, only the essential phrases required for a routine physical exam are provided here.

CHEST PAIN

Heart Disease	*Enfermedad Del Corazón*
Heart Failure	*Falla Cardiaca/Del Corazón*
Heart Broken	*Muerto De Pena*
Heart Attack	*Ataque Al Corazón*
Heart Murmur	*Soplo Del Corazón*
Heart Burn/Acid Stomach	*Acedía/Agruras*

RADIATION/LOCATION

Where do you feel (the pain)?	*¿Dónde siente (el dolor)?*
Point to/Show me where the pain is (with one finger).	*Apunta/Enséñame dónde le duele (con un dedo).*
Where does it run (the pain, the feeling)?	*¿Dónde corre (el dolor, la sensación)?*
...Arm, Back, Jaw, Shoulder	*...Brazo, Espalda, Quijada, Hombros*
Have you had any hurt/injury to your chest recently?	*¿Ha tenido algun lastimo/ daño a su pecho recientemente?*

QUALITY/QUANTITY

Have you had this problem before?	*¿Ha tenido este problema antes?*
Has it been always like this?	*¿Ha sido siempre así?*
Has it been the same as before?	*¿Ha sido igual que antes?*
What kind of pain (have you)?	*¿Qué clase de dolor (tiene)?*
Began slowly or rapidly?	*¿Empezó despacio o rápído?*

Boring	*Penetrante*	Pressure	*Con Presión*
Burning	*Que Quema/ Ardiente*	Referred	*Referido*
Continuous	*Continuo*	Ripping	*Rasgante*
Cramping	*Calambre*	Sharp	*Agudo*
Deep	*Hondo*	Shooting	*Punzante*
Dull	*Sordo*	Suffocation	*Sofocación*
Gripping	*Resgante*	Tearing	*Desgarrante*
Heavy	*Pesado*	That Moves	*Que Se Mueve*
Intense	*Intensivo*	Throbbing	*Pulsante*
Intermittent	*Intermitente*	Tightness	*Tirantez*
Light/Moderate	*ligero/Moderado*	Severe	*Severo/Fuertes*

PROVOCATIVE/PALLIATIVE

What makes it worse?	¿Qué lo hace peor?
What makes it better?	¿Qué lo hace mejor?
It is worse when...?	¿Está peor cuándo...?
...Walking/At Work	...Camina/Trabaja
...Agitation	...Ajitación/De Ajita
...Feel Very Stressed	...Siente Mucho Tensión
...Before/After You Eat	...Antes/Después De Comer
...You Are Cold/Hot	...Estas Frío/Caliente
It is better when...	¿Está mejor cuándo...?
...You're In Bed	...Está En La Cama?
...You're Resting	...Está Descansando?

SYMPTOMS

Have you.../Are you...?	¿Tiene.../Está usted...?
...Chest Pain Or Angina	...Dolor De Pecho o Angina De Pecho
...Palpitations	...Palpitaciónes
...Pain At Rest	...Dolores Al Descansar
...Swelling of the Hands, Face, Legs	...Hinchazón de las Manos, el Rostro, las Piernas
...Shortness Of Breath	...Corta La Respiración
...Nausea Or Vomiting	...Nausea o Vómito
...Sweaty	...Sudosoro
...Dizziness	...Mareos
...Weak Or Tired	...Débil O Cansado

RISK FACTORS

Do you have or have you had (at any time)...?	¿Tiene o ha tenido (alguna vez)...?
Anyone in your family have or every had...	¿Alguno de su familia estuvo o ha tenido...?
...Diabetes (DM)	...Diabetes
...Heart Attack (MI)	...Ataque Al Corazón
...Heart Disease	...Enfermedades De Corazón
...High Blood Pressure (HTN)	...Alta Presión
...Stroke	...Apoplejía/ Derrame (Cerebral)

...High Cholesterol	...Alto Colesterol
Smoke? How many packs a day (week)?	*¿Fuma? ¿Cuantos paquetes al dia (semana)?*
Drink? How many bottles a day (week)?	*¿Toma? ¿Cuantos botellas al dia (semana)?*

NITROGLYCERIN (NTG)

Do you have to take a medicine for the heart?	*¿Tiene usted que tomar tableta para el corazón?*
The tablet relieves the pain?	*¿La tableta alivia el dolor?*
Under the tongue?	*¿Debajo de la lengua?*
A white tablet, tiny, under the tongue?	*¿Tableta blanca, chiquita, debajo de la lengua?*

Cultural Note: You may hear the word "dolorcitas" which is the dimunitive of "dolor." It means "little pains."

Most pronounciation in Spanish can be fudged, but you should get to know the sound of 'ñ' (the 'ny' sound in 'canyon'). Don't pronounce it as an 'n.' The phrase "Cuántos años tiene?" takes on a whole new (embarrassing) meaning.

HEADACHE

RADIATION/LOCATION

Where do you feel? (the pain)	*¿Dónde siente (el dolor)?*
Point to where the pain is (with one finger).	*Apunte dónde le dolor (con un dedo).*
Where does it run (the pain, the feeling)?	*¿Dónde corre (el dolor, la sensación)?*
...Back, Jaw, Shoulder	*...Espalda, Quijada, Hombros*

QUALITY/DURATION

How long have you had (this problem)?	*¿Cuánto tiempo ha tenido (este problema)?*
For how long? (Duration)	*¿Por cuánto tiempo?*
Have you had this problem before?	*¿Ha tenido este problema antes?*
Has it been always like this?	*¿Ha sido siempre así?*
What kind of pain (have you)?	*¿Qué clase de dolor (tiene)?*
Began slowly or rapidly?	*¿Empezó despacio o rápído?*

Continuous	*Continuo*	**Moderate**	*Moderado*
Deep	*Hondo*	**Pressure**	*Con Presión*
Heavy	*Pesado*	**Severe**	*Severo/Fuertes*
Intense	*Intensivo*	**Sharp**	*Agudo*
Intermittent	*Intermitente*	**Throbbing**	*Pulsante*
Light	*Ligero*	**Tightness**	*Tirantez*

TIME ASSOCIATIONS

For how long have you each pain?	*¿Por cuánto tiempo tiene cada dolor?*
How much time between the pains?	*¿Cuánto tiempo entre los dolores?*
When have you more pain?	*¿Cuándo tiene más dolor?*
When have you less pain?	*¿Cuándo tiene menos dolor?*
...When you get up in the morning	*...Cuando se levante por la mañana*
...In The Morning	*...En La Mañana*
...Noon "Middle Day"	*...Medio Dias*
...The Afternoon	*...La Tarde*
...At Night	*...De Noche*

It occurs at the same hour
  every day?

Empiesa a la misma hora cada dia?

SYMPTOMS

Have you.../Are you...?	*¿Tiene.../Está usted...?*
...Nausea Or Vomiting	*...Nausea O Vómito*
...Sweaty	*...Sudosoro*
...Blackouts	*...Vísion Negras*
...Bright Lights Painful To Eyes	*...Luz Brilliante causa le duele a los ojos*
...Blindness	*...Ceguera*
...Fainting Spells	*...Desmayos*
...Blurred Vision (At Times)	*...Vista Borrosa (A Veces)*
...Tearing Of The Eyes	*...Le Lagrimean Los Ojos*
...Stuffy Nose	*...La Nariz Tapada*
...Neck Pain Or Feel Stiff/ Hard	*...Dolor De Cuello O Siente Tieso/Duro*
...Dizziness	*...Mareos*
...Hallucinations	*...Alucinaciónes*

CAUSATIVE FACTORS

What is the cause of your headaches?	*¿Qué es lo qué causa el dolor de su cabeza?*
...Menses	*...La Regla*
...Birth Control Pills	*...Pastillas Anticonceptivas*
...Stress/Anxiety	*...Tensión/Ansiedad*
...Hunger	*...Hambre*
...No Sleep	*...No Dormir*
...Too Much Sleep	*...Dormir demasiado*
...Fatigue	*...Fatiga*
...Work	*...Trebaje*
...Bright Lights	*...Luz Fuerte/Luz Brilliante*
...Foods	*...Comidas*
...Chocolate	*...Chocolate*
...Cheese	*...Queso*
...Alcohol	*...Alcohol*
...Salt/MSG	*...Sal/MSG*

...Bacon (as an example of nitrates)   ...*Tocino*

Is bright light painful to your eyes?   *¿Le duele la luz fuertes a los ojos?*

OBSTETRICS & GYNECOLOGY

- **OB/GYN HISTORY OUTLINE**
- **OB SCREEEENING**
- **PREGNANCY HISTORY**
- **THE GYN EXAM**
- **LABOR & DELIVERY**
- **POST PARTUM/POST-OP**
- **BIRTH CONTROL COUNSELING**

OB/GYN HISTORY:

Menstruation: Menarche, LMP, Menstrual Pattern (interval, amount, duration, intermittent bleeding, dysmenorrhea, PMS symptoms).

OB: Gravidity/Parity. Describe each pregnancy (date, outcome, complications) Use TPAL (Term babies, Pre-term babies, Abortions [spontaneous or induced], Living children) system to numerically score gravidity and parity.

Birth Control: Current method, sexually active, past methods used (complications, why changed), sterilizations.

Sexual History: Sexual orientation, sexual patterns, dyspareunia, sexual problems.

Infertility: difficultly becoming pregnant. Medical evaluation or treatment.

PAP: Last pap, usual frequency, any abnormal results.

Infection: Vaginal discharges (onset, pattern, color, odor, symptoms-itching/pain), prior vaginal infections (type, frequency, treatment of self and partner), STD's (herpes, gonorrhea, chlamydia, condylomata), PID.

Pelvic Relaxation: Prolapse, vaginal splinting, urinary retention/incontinence.

Breast: Masses, discharge, pain, problems, FHx breast cancer.

Social: Marital status, educational background, father of baby (FOB) participation, drugs (especially in 1st trimester), seat belt use.

(Please see Review of Systems for a review of Sexual History)

OPENING LINES

Do you have a friend who speaks English (with you)?	*¿Tiene un amigo que habla ingles (con usted)?*
I am just learning to speak Spanish...	*Yo estoy apenas aprendiendo a hablar Español...*
I don't speak good Spanish...	*No hablo muy bien español...*
I'm reading from a list of questions...	*Estoy leyendo de un questionario varias preguntas...*
That I need to know about you...	*Que necesito saber de usted...*
Please answer "yes" or "no" to my questions...	Por favor conteste "si" o "no" a mis preguntas...
Please answer my questions slowly...	Por favor conteste mis preguntas despacio...
Understand?	*¿Entiende?*
Write down the date...	*Escriba la fecha...*
Write down the number...	*Escriba el numero...*

OB SCREENING

Hello. How are you?	*¡Hola! ¿Cómo esta?*
In what way can I help you?	*¿En que le puedo ayudar?*
Do you have your (blue), (green), (red), (yellow) card?	*¿Tiene su tarjeta (azul), (verde), (roja), (amarillo)?*
Are you pregnant?	*¿Está Embarazada/Encinta?*
Are you going to have a baby?	*¿Va a tener un bebé?*
Do you have any papers to give the doctor?	*¿Tiene algunes papeles para darle al doctor?*
We are very busy...	*Estamos muy ocupados...*
We will see you as soon as we can...	*Lo veremos lo más pronto que podamos...*
Everyone must wait their turn...	*Todo tiene que esperar su turno...*

MENSTRUAL menarche, menstrual triad (cycle, duration, dysmenorrhea) vaginal discharge (color, amount, odor, consistency, pain, itching), number of pregnancies, number of deliveries, number of abortions, number of living, problem in delivery, last PAP (date & result), menopausal symptoms.

Dizziness	*Mareo*
Labor/Delivery	*El Parto*
Short/Long	*Corto/Largo*
The Menstrual Period	*La Regla/Menstruación*
Miscarriages	*Mal-partos*
Abortions	*Abortos*
Still Births "Born Dead"	*Niños Nacidos Muertos*
Pregnancy	*El Embarazo*
Pregnant (Euphemisms)	*Encinta/Embarazada*
What date?	*¿Qué fecha?*

At what age did the periods begin?	*¿A qué edad tuvo su primer regla?*
What age did you start to mensturate?	*¿A qué edad empezo su regla/menstraccion?*
When was your last period?	*¿Cuándo fue su ultima regla?*
For how many days duration?	*¿Por cuántos dias dura?*
How many days do you bleed?	*¿Por cuántos días sangra?*
How many days between your periods?	*¿Cuánto diás entre sus reglas?*
Did you have a normal period?	*¿Tuvo una regla normal?*
Do you have pains with your menses?	*¿Tiene dolor con sus reglas?*
Any unusual bleeding between periods?	*¿Algun sangrado inusual entre reglas/periodos?*
You bleed a lot? With pain?	*¿Sangra mucho? ¿Con dolor?*
Are you passing clots? Very large?	*¿Pasas coágulos? ¿Muy grandes?*
Do you have vaginal discharge/secretions?	*¿Tiene flujós/desechos vaginales?*
Of what color? A little? A lot?	*¿De qué color? ¿Poco? ¿Mucho?*
Bad smelling? Nauseating/ Smelly?	*¿Mal olor? ¿Apesta/ Maloliente?*
Thick or not thick?	*¿Espeso o no espeso?*
A lot of itching? Pain?	*¿Mucho comezón? ¿Dolor?*
How many total pregnancies?	*¿Cuántos embarazos en total?*

How many children have you?	*¿Cuántos niños tiene usted?*
How many children living?	*¿Cuántos niños vivos?*
How many children dead?	*¿Cuántos niños muertos?*
How many miscarriages?	*¿Cuántos malpartos?*
The weight of the last baby?	*¿El peso del último bebé/niño?*
The last delivery...	*¿El último parto...?*
...Short or Long?	*...Corto o Largo?*
...Have any problems?	*...Tuvo algunos problemas?*
When was your last Cancer/ Pap (Papanicolado) test?	*¿Cuándo fue su ultima prueba de cáncer/Pap (Papanicolado)?*
Do you have the urge to vomit in the morning?	*¿Tiene usted ganas de vomitar en la mañana?*

Spanish Note: It's common if you're just learning Spanish to substitute in conversation an English word for a Spanish word but pronounced with a Spanish accent. This actually works with many words (e.g. Diarrhea, Infection, etc.) and the patient may get the 'jist' of what is meant. However, if you are "embarrassed," don't say, "Mi es Embarazada" otherwise you will be admitting you are pregnant.

PRENATAL DROP-IN - INITIAL QUESTIONS

Is this your first baby?	*¿Es su primer bebé?*
Is this your first pregnancy?	*¿Es su primer embarazo?*
When is your baby going to be born?	*¿Cuándo va a nacer su niño?*
Approximate date of delivery?	*¿Fecha aproximada del parto?*
Why did you come to the hospital/clinic?	*Por qué ha venido a la hospital/clinica?*
Have you been going to clinic?	*¿Ha venido a la clinica?*
How many times? Which clinic?	*¿Cuántas veces? ¿Cuál clinica?*
When was the last time you went to clinic? What date?	*¿Cuándo fue la última vez que fuiste a la clinica? ¿Qué fecha?*
In what month (of your pregnancy) did you go to the doctor to begin your care?	*¿En qué mes (de su embarazo) vio al doctor para empezar el cuidado de maternidad?*
The last delivery - short or long?	*El último parto - ¿corto o largo?*
Are you taking your vitamins and iron?	*¿Estas tomando los vitaminas y hierro?*
I need to examine you...	*Necesito examinarla...*
I need to have a sample of blood/urine.	*Necesito una muestra de su sangre/orina.*

Cultural Note: "*Las partes*" (The private "parts") can be used to examine the breasts and genital system. It is important to inform your female patients <u>before</u> you begin to examine their breasts.

PREGNANCY HISTORY

How old are you "have many years have you?"	¿Cuantos años tiene?
Your normal weight is?	¿Su peso es normal?
How much do you weigh?	¿Cuánto pesa?
How much weight have you gained (in pounds)?	¿Cuánto peso ha subido (en libras)?
How many pregnancies have you had (in total)?	¿Cuántos embarazos ha tenido usted (en total)?
How many children were nine months (forty weeks)?	¿Cuantos niños fueron nueve meses (cuarenta semanas)?
How many children were premature? (Less then thirty-seven weeks?)	¿Cuantos niños fueron prematuros? (¿Menos de treinta y siete semanas?)
How many abortions have you had?	¿Cuantos abortos ha tenido?
Have you ever had a miscarriage?	¿Ha tenido un malparte?
How many miscarriages?	¿Cuantos mal-partos?
Have you ever had a stillborn?	¿Ha tenido un niño qué nació muerto?
How many children are living?	¿Cuantos niños están vivos?
After birth, any problems with the children?	¿Después de nacer, habia algunos problemas con los niños?
Have you taken pill (contraceptives) during the past (six)/(twelve) months?	¿Has estado tomando pastillas (anticonceptivas) durante los últimos (seis)/ (doce) meses?
What was the first day of your last menstrual period?	
Your period is regular or irregular?	¿Sus regla (menstruación) es regular o irregular?
When did you have your last period?	¿Cuándo fue se última regla?
Did you have a normal period?	¿Tuvo una regla normal?
Was it a normal period?	¿Fue esta regla normal?
When you had the period before the last period, was it normal or abnormal?	¿Cuando fue la regla antes de la última regla, fue normal o anormal?

Have you had a pregnancy test? Was it positive or negative? What date?	¿Ha tenido una test (prueba) de embarazo? ¿Fue positiva o negativa? ¿Qué fecha?
Your First, Second, Third, Fourth, Fifth, Sixth, Seventh, Eighth pregnancy/birth...	Sus Primero, Segundo, Tercero, Cuarto, Quinto, Sexto, Séptimo, Octavo embarazo/parto...
...When was it? (What month, what year?)	...Cuando fué? (¿Qué mes, qué año?)
...How many months was it? (Nine months, full term, premature)	...Cuantos meses tenia? (Nueve meses/ términado/ prematuro)
...Was it a boy or a girl?	...Fué niño o niña?
...How much did your child weigh? (Pounds and ounces or Kilograms and grams)	...Cuanto pesó el niño? (Libras y onzas o Kilos y gramos)
...Is the child alive?	...Está vivo el niño?
...The child was born by Cesarean or it came naturally (vaginally)?	...El niño nació por Cesárea o por vias naturales (vaginales)?
Why was it Cesarean?	¿Por qué fué Cesárea?
...High blood pressure	...Alta Presion de sangre
...Bleeding	...Sangrado
...Large Baby	...Bebé Más Grande
...Narrow Pelvis	...Estrecha De La Pelvis
...Fatigue	...Fatiga
...Slow Labor	...Parto Lento
...The head was too large	...La cabeza era demasiado grande
...It was a repeat	...Fué repetición
...The baby had problems	...El niño tenia problemas
The baby came sitting (breech)?	¿El niño vino sentado?
Head down (vertex)?	¿Cabeza abajo?
They had to use forceps?	¿Le tuvieron que usar forceps?
Have you had ectopic pregnancies? (Pregnancies in the tubes?)	¿Ha tenido embarazos ectopicos? (¿Embarazos en los trompas/ tubos?)
Have you had induced abortions (by a Doctor)?	¿Ha tenido abortos inducidos (por un Médico)?

Your child born dead or died after delivery?	¿Su niño nacio muerto o se murio despues de del parto?
You child had neurologic problems/ mentally retarded?	¿Su niño tiene problemas neurologicos/son retrasado mentales?
You child had jaundice (yellow skin)?	Su nino ha tenido ictericia o piel amarilla?
Your child has genetic disease? Down's?	Sus niño tiene enfermedades geneticas? ¿Minos mongolicos?

Do you have allergies to medicines or foods?	¿Tiene alérgicas a medicinas o comidas/almientos?
Do you have an allergy to...?	¿Tiene alérgia a...?
...Penicillin	...Penicilina
...Aspirin	...Aspirina
...Anesthesia	...Anestesia
...Antibiotics	...Antibióticos
...Other Medicines	...Otra Medicinas

Do you have or have you had (at any time)...?	*¿Tiene o ha tenido (alguna vez)...?*
...Candidiasis	...Moniliasis
...Canker Sores	...Postemilla
...Chancre	...Chancro
...Chlamydia	...Clamidia
...Condyloma	...Condiloma
...Gonorrhea	...Gonorrea
...Herpes (Genital)	...Herpes Genital
...Oral Lesions	...Fuegos En La Boca
...Syphilis	...Sífilis
...Trichomonas	...Tricomonas
...Warts (Genital)	...Verruga Genital

Do you have or have you had (at any time)...?	*¿Tiene o ha tenido (alguna vez)...?*
Problems with...	*Problemas con...*
...lungs	...los pulmones
...kidneys	...los riñones
...heart	...el corazón
...thyroid	...la tiroides

Do you bleed easily?	*¿Sangrar fácilmente?*
Do you bruise easily?	*¿Fácilmente se moretea?*
Do you have any other medical problems?	*¿Tiene otra problemas medicos?*
...Bleeding tendency?	*...Tendencia a sangrar?*
...Diabetes/Hepatitis	*...Diabetes/Hepatitis*
...Hemophilia?	*...Hemofilia?*
...Hemorrhage	*...Hemorragia (Sangrado)*
...Hypertension	*...Alta Presión (De Sangre)*
...Hypertension during pregnancy?	*...Alta Presión (De Sangre) durante el embarazo?*
...Infections in the kidneys	*...Infecciónes de los riñones*
...Infections in the urine	*...Infecciónes de la orina?*
...Nose bleeds?	*...Sangramiento por la nariz?*
...Phlebitis?	*...Flebitis?*
...Problems getting pregnant	*...Problemas en quedar embarazada?*
...Problems with anesthesia?	*...Problemas con anestesia?*
...Problems with the thyroid?	*...Problemas con la tiroides?*
...Rheumatic Fever	*...Fiebre Reumática*
...Surgery of the uterus?	*...De cirugia en the matriz?*
...Tuberculosis	*...Tuberculosis*
...With your cervix (the neck of the uterus) or with your uterus?	*...con su cerviz (el cuello de la matriz) o con su matriz?*
Have you had (any)...?	*¿Ha tenido (algunas)...?*
...Operations? For what?	*...Operaciónes? ¿De qué?*
...They took out your tonsils?	*...¿Le sacaron las amígdala/ glandulas salivares?*
...They took out your appendix?	*...¿Le sacaron la apéndice?*
Smoke?	*¿Fuma?*
How many packs a day (week)?	*¿Cuántos paquetes al dia (semana)?*
Drink?	*¿Toma?*
Every Day? ("all the days")	*¿Todos los días?*
How many a day?	*¿Cuántas al dia?*

How many bottles a day (week)?	¿Cuántas botellas al dia (semana)?
...Alcohol	...Alcohol
...Beer	...Cerveza
...Wine	...Vino "Vee-No"
...Whiskey	...Whiskey "We-Ski"

Do you use or have you used (at any time)...?	¿Usa o ha usado (alguna vez)...?
...Intravenous Drugs	...Drogas Intravenosas
...Cocaine	...Cocaína
...Crack	...Crac ("Crak")
...Heroin	...Heroína
...Marijuana	...Marijuana
...Methadone	...Metadona
...Opium	...Opio
...Or Any Others Drug	...O Alguna Otra Droga

Do you have illnesses in your family (like)...	Hay enfermedades en su familia (como)...
...Cancer (of the breast)	...Cáncer (de los pechos)
...Twins or Multiple Births	...Gemelos o Partos Múltiples
...Hypertension during pregnancy?	...Alta Presión (De Sangre) durante el embarazo?
...Hypertension/ Toxemia	...Alta Presión (De Sangre)/ Toxemia
...Diabetes/Hepatitis	...Diabetes/Hepatitis
...Asthma	...Asma
...Hemophilia?	...Hemofilia?

PREGNANCY CHECK-UP VISIT

Have you had any problems with this pregnancy?	¿Ha tenido algunos problemas con este embarazo?
Have you had any bleeding?	¿Ha sangrado alguna ves?
Are you passing clots? Very large?	¿Pasas coágulos? ¿Muy grandes?
Have you had any infections? Of where?	¿Ha tenido alguna infeccions? ¿De qué?
Have you had pain at urination (dysuria)?	¿Ha tenido dolores al orinar?
Do you have the urge to urinate frequently (often)?	¿Tiene ganas de orinar muy frecuente (muy amenudo)?
Have you spots/stars in front of the eyes?	¿Ha tenido manchas/estrellas enfrente de los ojos?
Any problems with your vision?	¿Algun problema con su vision/vista?
Have you had severe headaches?	¿Ha tenido dolores fuertes en la cabeza?
How many times in a week?	¿Cuántas veces en una semana?
Have you had nausea or vomiting?	¿Ha tenido náuseas o vómito?
Have you dizziness?	¿Ha tenido mareo?
Have you been vomiting?	¿Ha estado vomitando?
Have you had hypertension?	¿Ha tenido altá presion?
Have you had swelling of both hands, face, or legs?	¿Se le han hinchado las manos, el rostro (la cara), o las piernas?
Can you use/wear your rings?	¿Puede usar/ponerse sus anillos?
Since when have you been swollen?	¿Desde cuando han estado hinchados?
Do you tire easily?	¿Se cansa facil?
Do you have or have you had difficulty breathing?	¿Tiene o ha tenido dificultad para respirar?
After work? When you lie down?	¿Después de trabajar? ¿Cuándo se acuesta?
Have you palpitations of the heart?	¿Ha tenido palpitaciones de corazón?
Have you had diarrhea? Constipation?	¿Ha tenido diarrea? ¿Estreñimiento?
Have you had any seizures?	¿Ha tenido o le dan ataques?

Have you had bleeding?	*¿Ha sangrado?*
Are you bleeding?	*¿Esta sangrando?*
Was the color pink or bright red?	*¿Fue del color rosa o rojo claro?*
How much blood...?	*¿Cuánta sangre...?*
...A Cupful?	*...Una Taza?*
...A Tablespoonful?	*...Una Cucharada?*
...A Teaspoonful?	*...Una Cucharadita?*
Have you taken birth control pills in the past year?	*¿A tomado pildoras para control de natalidad el año pasado?*
Have you taken contraceptive pills (for "no pregnancy")?	*¿A tomado usted pildoras anticonceptivas (para "no embarazarse")?*

Cultural Note: Without trying to make broad generalizations, I have found my female Latin American & Mexican patients to be very modest regarding sexual relations. Simply *asking* questions pertaining to sexual matters or birth control can cause embarrassment and a frank refusal to answer any questions.

Often you may find your Mexican/Latino patient covering her face with a sheet or towel (or dress!) during a pelvic examination. This is an extremely private affair for your patient – regardless if the physician is male for female. You should be aware that what we consider routine medical care in the U. S. can be extremely distressing to your patients.

OB/GYN EXAMINATION

For additional positioning commands, see "Physical Exam" section.

My name is _____...	*Me llamo _____...*
I am going to examine you...	*Voy a examinarla...*
I need to make an exam internally...	*Necisito hacerle un examen interno...*
Sit here...	*Sientese aquí...*
Lie down...	*Acuestese...*
...Here	*...Aquí*
...On Your Back	*...En Su Espalda*
...Face Up ("Mouth-Up")	*...Boca Arriba*
...Face Down ("Mouth-Down")	*...Boca Debajo*
...On Your Left/Right Side	*...De Lado Izquierda/Derecha*
Place/Put your feet in the stirrups...	*Ponga los pies en los estribas...*
Open/Relax your legs...	*Abra/Relaje las piernas...*
Bend your knees...	*Doble las rodillas...*
Put together the feet...	*Junte los pies...*
Relax your body...	*Descanse el cuerpo...*
Left your hips/lift yourself...	*Levante las caderas/ levantese..*
Move yourself (until the edge of the table)... More...	*Muevase (hasta la orilla de la mesa)... Más...*
This is going to hurt a little...	*Esto va a doler muy poco...*
It is a protection against cancer...	*Es una despensa contra el cáncer...*
Pain when I push?	*¿Duele cuando yo empujó?*
Do you have pain? Now? Where?	*¿Tiene dolor? ¿Ahorita? ¿Dónde?*
Don't push...	*No empuje...*
Raise your legs...	*Levante las piernas...*
Breathe by the mouth...	*Respire por la boca...*
The baby is not coming today.	*El niño no sale hoy...*
The baby will come soon...	*El niño saldra pronto...*

ADVICE TO NON-ADMITTED LABOR PATIENTS
(AMBULATE IN THE HOSPITAL OR SENT HOME)

You are not going to deliver.	*No ira dar parto hoy.*
You will not be admitted to the hospital.	*No la vamos a admitir al hospital.*
You can go to your home.	*Se puede ir a su casa.*
You are in the first part of labor.	*Esta en la primera parte del parto.*
Go home and lie down.	*Vayase a casa y acuestese.*
Stay here in the hospital and walk for ___ hours.	*Quedese aquí en al hospital y camine por ___ horas.*
You have to walk one hour then return.	*Tiene qué caminar/andar una hora y luego regresar.*
Return in ___ hours.	*Regrese en ___ horas.*
Return to the clinic when or if your water bag ruptures.	*Regrese a la clinica cuando o si se reviente la bolsa de agua.*
Or when the pains are stronger and every ___ minutes.	*O cuándo sus dolores estan más fuertes y cada ___ minutos.*
If you are not better in __days	*Si usted no se mejora en __ días*
See your private doctor or return here...	*Vea a su propio doctor o regrese aquí...*

THE LABOR

When did the pains begin?	*¿Cuándo empezaron/comenzaron los dolores?*
Did you rupture/burst the water bag?	*¿Se le rompio/revento la bolsa de agua?*
Did you brake the water bag?	*¿Usted roto la bolsa de agua?*
At what time did it break?	*¿A qué hora se le revento?*
How much water lost? Down the legs?	*¿Cuánta agua pérdio? ¿Se le bajo por las piernas?*
How often are your pains (in minutes)?	*¿Cada cuanto le dan los dolores (en minutos)?*
At what hour did they become regular?	*¿A qué hora fueron regulares?*
With what frequency when they became regular?	*¿Con qué frecuencia fueron cuando empezaron regulares?*
With what frequency are they now?	*¿Con qué frecuencia estan ahorita?*
For what duration?	*¿Por cuánto duran?*
Breath only when you have the pains.	*Respire solamente cuando tenga los dolores.*
Push with the pains (contractions).	*Empuja con los dolores (contracciónes).*
Call when you have the next pain.	*Llame cuando tenga el proximo dolor.*
Breath with this mask. It is oxygen.	*Respire con esta mascara. Esto es oxigeno.*
You are going to the operating room.	*Va a la sala de operaciones.*
I'm going to look.	*Voy a ver.*
The baby is not coming today...	*El niño no sale hoy...*
The baby will come soon...	*El niño saldra pronto...*

SOME SIMPLE LABOR NURSING INSTRUCTIONS

You are going to stay in the hospital.	*Se va a quedar en el hospital.*
The doctor wants you to stay in the hospital.	*El doctor quiere qué se quede en el hospital.*
Is someone waiting for you?	*¿Esta alguien esperando por usted?*
Sign here… to receive your clothes.	*Firme aquí… para recibir su ropa.*
We are going to take an X-ray…	*Va a tomar una radiografia…*
Do not lock the door…	*Use la cerradura en la puerta…*
Call when you have to use the bedpan…	*Llame cuando tenga qué usar el basin…*
I need to have a sample of blood/urine.	*Necesito una muestra de su sangre/orina.*
You need a bedpan?	*¿Necesita el basin?*
Have you urinated? ("Have you made pee?")	*¿Ha orinado? ("¿Ha hecho pipi?")*
Since when have you not urinated?	*¿Desde cuando no ha orinado?*
Have you finished?	*¿Ha terminado?*
Are you urinating enough?	*¿Esta orinado bastante?*
I am going to give you an enema (suppository)…	*Voy a darle una lavativo (supositorio)…*
You have to use this towel to clean your rectum, from the front towards the back, before you can give me a sample of urine…	*Usted tiene que usar esta toalla para limpiar su recto, desde el frente hacia atrás, antes de que me dé una muestra de orina…*
Come with me…	*Venga con migo…*
You have to rest in bed…	*Usted tiene que descansar en cama…*
I have to clean your…	*Tengo que limpiarle su(s)…*
Do you want more…	*¿Quiere más…*
…Blankets	*…Frazadas*
…Food	*…Comidas*
…Medicine for pain	*…Medicinas para dolor*
…Water	*…Agua*
…Light	*…Luz*
…Paper	*…Papel*
…Pain Killer	*…Analgésico*

THE DELIVERY

Breath with the pains...	*Respire con los dolores...*
Breath like this. (demonstrate for the patient)	*Respire así.*
Pant	*Jadee*
Blow	*Sopla*
I need to examine you...	*Necesito examenarla...*
Place/Put your foot in this stirrup...	*Ponga el pie en esta estriba...*
Open/Relax your legs (knees)...	*Abre/Relaje los piernas (rodillas)...*
Don't touch here. Keep the hands under the towels/ sheets/ blankets.	*No toque aquí! Deje las manos debajo de las toallas/ sabanas/ Frazadas*
Push with the pains...	*Empuje con los dolores...*
Push! Stronger! ("More severe")...	*¡Empuje! ¡Más fuerte!...*
Again ("Another time")... For 10 seconds... One, two, three...	*Otra vez... Por diez segundos... Uno, dos, tres...*
Push with your rectum... (As if going to the bathroom...)	*Empuje con su recto... (Cómo si va ir al baño...)*
Hands on your knees...	*Manos en las rodillas...*
Pull (grab) your knees, push with your rectum...	*Tire (agarre) sus rodillas, empuje con su recto...*
No more pushing...	*No empuje más...*
A little needle stick...	*Un piquete agudo...*
This is anesthesia... It makes you feel sleepy...	*Este es anestesia... La hara sentirse dormida...*
I'm going to give medicine for the pain...	*Le voy a dar medicina para el dolor...*
I need to make a small cut to make more room for the baby...	*Nesesito hocerle un pequeño corte para hacer mas espacio para el niño...*
Congratulations!	*¡Felicidades!*
It's a boy! It's a little man!	*Es un niño! Es un hombrecito!*
It's a girl! It's a little woman!	*Es una niña! Es una mujercita!*
Dad, please cut the cord...	*Papá, por favor corte el cordon*

Your baby weighs ___ pounds and ___ ounces...	*Su bebé pesa ___ libras y ___ onzas...*
Good Luck! Much Luck!	*¡Buena suerte! ¡Muchas suerte!*
Do you have a name for the baby?	*¿Tiene un nombre para el bebé?*
Much bleeding, madame...	*Mucho sangrado, señora...*
I need to push on your uterus...	*Necisito empujar su matriz...*
You have a lot of bleeding. I have to give a message on your abdomen/ belly/ uterus.	*Tiene mucho sangrado. Tengo que darle masaje en su abdomen/ panza/ matriz.*
You will need sutures...	*Necesitara puntadas...*
I am going to put a few stitches in your vagina...	*Voy a darle unas puntadas en la vagina...*
The stiches will dissolve by themselves.	*Las puntadas se disolverán solas.*
Your baby has some medical problems...	*Su bebé tiene unos problemas médicos...*
We will call a pediatrician and a translator...	*Llamaremos a pediatrico y un intérprete...*

OB/GYN POST-OP/POST PARTUM

Do you have hunger/thirst?	*¿Tiene hambre/sed?*
Have you defecated after delivery?	*¿Ha defecado después de el parto?*
Have you gone to the bathroom (after delivery)?	*¿Ha ido al baño (después del parto)?*
How many hours ago?	*¿Cuándas horas antes?*
Did you get up? Walked?	*¿Se ha levantado? ¿Caminado?*
Do you have headache or spots before your eyes?	*¿Tiene dolor en su cabeza o manchas enfrente de sus ojos?*
Do you have pain in your...	*¿Tiene dolor en sus...?*
...Breasts or Head?	*...Pechos o Cabeza?*
...Heart or Lungs?	*...Corazón o Pulmones?*
...Abdomen or Legs?	*...Abdomen o Piernas?*
Do you have any contractions ("pains")?	*¿Tiene contracciónes ("dolores")?*
I need to make a quick exam.	*Necesito hacer un examen rapido.*
Pain when I push?	*¿Duele cuando le empujó?*
I need to feel your abdomen.	*Necesito sentir su abdomen.*
I need to listen to your heart and lungs.	*Necesito escuchar a su corazón y pulmones.*
Your bleeding... a little or a lot?	*¿Esta sangrando... poquito o mucho?*
I need to check the bleeding in your "parts" (genitals).	*Necesito checar/revisar el sangrado en sus partes (genitales)*
You can have no sexual relations for six weeks.	*No tenga relaciónes (sexuales) por seis semanas.*
You need to return to clinic in (two)/(six) weeks.	*Necesita regresar a la clinica en (dos)/(seis) semanas*
You must take your baby to the pediatrician in (1) week.	*Necesita llevar a su bebé al pedíatra en una semana.*
For your baby - the bottle, the breasts, or both?	*Para su bebé - ¿la botella, el pecho, o los dos?*
Do you know what a circumcision is? Do you want one? (For your baby?)	*¿Sabe lo que es una circumcision? ¿Quiere una? (¿Para su bebé?)*
You can go home today (after lunch). In the afternoon.	*Puede irse a la casa hoy (después de almuerzo). En la tarde.*

ORAL CONTRACEPTIVE PILLS (OCP'S) - BIRTH CONTROL

PRIOR CONTRACEPTION

Do you use contraception?	¿Usa usted contraceptivos?
What kind of birth control have you been using...?	¿Qué clase de control de nacimiento ha usado...?
...Condoms	...Condoms
...Contraceptive Foam	...Espuma Anticonceptivas
...Contraceptive Pills	...Pastillas Anticonceptivas
...IUD (Intra-Uterine Device)	...El Apartato/Dispositivo Intra-uterino (D.I.U.)
...Diaphragm	...Diafragma
Had you any problems (with the pills)?	¿Tiene problemas (con las pastillas)?

ABSOLUTE/HIGH RISK CONTRAINDICATIONS

Have you used contraceptive pills before?	¿Ha usada usted anteriormente pildoras anticonceptivas?
Did you have much problems?	¿Tuvo usted muchos problemas?
Any heart attacks or stokes?	¿Algun ataque al corazón o derrame?
Any problems with your blood?	¿Algun problema con su sangre?
Any problems with blood clots (in the legs, lungs, or eyes)?	¿Algun problemas con coágulos de sangre? En sus piernas, pulmones, o ojos?
Any pain in the chest?	¿Algun dolor en el pecho?
Any cancers? (of the breast, cervix, vagina, or uterus?)	¿Algun cáncer, de los pechos, cerviz, vagina, o del utero?
Any unusual bleeding between periods?	¿Algun sangrado inusual entre periodos de menstruación?
Problems with your liver (any yellow pigment in the skin or eyes?)	¿Problemas con su hígado (algun pigmento amarillo en la piel o en los ojos)?
Any liver tumor?	¿Algun tumor en el hígado?
Are you pregnant?	¿Está embarazada?

MODERATE RISK CONTRAINDICATIONS

Do you have diabetes? (High blood sugar?)	¿Tiene usted diabetes? (Alta azúcar en la sangre?)

Do you have high blood pressure?	*¿Tiene alta presion?*
Do you suffer severe head aches (migraines) or seizures (convulsions)?	*¿Sufre usted de fuertes dolores de cabeza (migrañas) o ataques (convulsiones)?*
Do you have any heart or liver disease?	*¿Tiene alguna enfermedad del corazón o del hígado?*
Do you have any gall-bladder disease?	*¿Tiene algun problema con la vesicula biliar?*
Are you over 35 years old?	*¿Es usted mayor de 35 (treinta y cinco) años?*
Do you smoke?	*¿Fuma usted?*
Do you have any high cholesterol?	*¿Tiene alto colesterol?*
Do you have intense depressions?	*¿Tiene intensas depresiones?* or *¿Tiene depremidas intensas?*

RISKS

Taking these pills can increase the risk of suffering...	*Tomando esta pastillas podria aumentar el riesgo de sufrir...*
...Blood clots	*...Coágulos de sangre*
...Heart attack or stoke	*...Ataques al corazón o derrames*
...Gall bladder problems	*...Problemas en la vesicula biliar*
...Tumors in the liver	*...Tumor en el hígado*

SIDE EFFECTS

These pills have side effects, like...	*Estas pastillas tienen otros efectos, como...*
...Bleeding between menses	*...Sangrar entre periodos de menstruación*
...Dark spots on the skin	*...Manchas oscuras en la piel*
...Swelling/Inflammation (of the wrists and ankles)	*...Hinchazón/Inflamacion (de las muñecas y tobillos)*
...Nausea & vomiting	*...Náusea y vómito*
...Headache	*...Dolor de cabeza*
...Rash	*...Salpullido*
...Depression	*...Depresión*
Most of these symptoms get better after 3 months...	*La mayoria de estos síntomas se mejorán después de 3 (tres) meses...*

If they remain after 3 months, call your doctor…	Si sigen/permanecer después de (3) tres meses, llame a su doctor…
If they are severe, call your doctor…	Si son muy intensos, llama a su doctor…

BREAST FEEDING (Controversial Topic)

For your baby - the bottle, the breasts, or both?	¿Para su bebé - la botella, el pecho, o los dos?
The pills contain hormones…	Las pildoras contienen hormonas…
The hormones will get into the milk…	Las hormonas se irán dentro de la leche…
This will not cause any injury to your baby…	Esto no le causaría ningún daño a sus bebé…
You may note your baby's breasts get larger…	Usted nota el pecho de su bebé más grande…
Or you may notice a yellowing of the skin…	O quizas notara la piel amarilla…
Your breasts may get smaller…	Sus pechos se podrian poner un poco pequeños…
And the amount of milk is going to be deminished…	Y su cantidad de leche va a disminuir…
But it should be enough for your baby…	Pero esto sería suficeinte para su bebé…

STARTING THERAPY

Do you want a prescription for OCP's ("for no prenancy")?	¿Quieres una receta por pastillos anticonceptivas ("para no embarazarse")?
I will give you some pills today…	Voy a darle algunas pastillas hoy…
I will give you a prescription for (3) packs more…	Voy a darle una receta para tres paquetes más…
You need to start taking these pills on a Sunday…	Necesita empezar a tomar estas pastillas en Domingo…
Start to take the pills on Sunday…	Comience a tomar las pastillas el Domingo…
Take one pill just when you go to bed…	Tome una pildora cuando vaya a acostarse…
Begin to take your pills after (2) weeks…	Comienze a tomar sus pastillas después de (2) dos semanas…

Your menses may be less than what is normal...	*Su regla/menstruación podria ser menor de cuando es normal...*
You may have less cramping...	*Usted podria tener menos calambres...*
Your menses should begin on a Tuesday or Wednesday...	*Su regla/menstruación deberia comenzar el Martes o Miercoles...*
If you forget to take (1) pill, take it immediately when you remember...	*Si usted olvida de tomar una pastilla, tomela immediatamente cuando lo recuerde...*
And take your usual pill before laying down to sleep...	*Y tome su pastilla usual antes de acostarse a dormir...*
If you forget to take (2) pills, take (2) pills at before laying down to sleep for (2) nights...	*Si usted olvida de tomar dos pastillas, tome dos pastillas antes de acostarse a dormir por dos noches...*

PEDIATRICS

- SCREENING QUESTIONS
- VOCABULARY
- NEWBORN EXAM
- DEVELOPMENTAL MILESTONES

<u>BRIEF WELL CHILD CHECK (WCC)</u> - modify for age

IDENTIFYING DATA: Age, race, sex, reason for visit, duration of any complaint

CONSTITUTIONAL SYMPTOMS: fevers, chills, emesis, cough, runny nose, diarrhea, constipation, recurrent infections

BIRTH HISTORY: Maternal **G:**(total pregnancies) **P:**(full term, pre-term, abortions, total living), duration of labor, Cesarean or vaginal delivery (NSVD), where born, gestational age, illness during pregnancy, complications. How many days in hospital before discharge for mother and infant.

FEEDS: bottle/breasts, amount, frequency

SLEEP: duration of daytime & nighttime sleep

STOOL: frequency, color, consistency

DEVELOPMENTAL: motor, language, social (Denver)

SAFETY: car seat use, smoke alarm in the home

HOME: total adults, children, any ill contacts, any smokers. Father of baby involved. Primary care giver.

VACCINATIONS/ALLERGIES: immunizations up to date (UTD), any adverse reactions, allergies to foods or medicines

PHYSICAL EXAM: General appearance, vital signs, skin, head, eyes, ears, nose, mouth, neck, heart, lungs, back, abdomen, hips, extremities, genitourinary, neurologic.

PLAN: WCC, anticipatory guidance, immunizations, supplements: (iron, flouride, multivitamin), next appointment date.

NOTE: "Personality" is a good general screening question at the first two WCC visits. *Children in their first few weeks have no personality*, and the answer the mother gives may reflect upon her acceptance and/or understanding of her child. (Once a young mother of a healthy 2 month old told me she believed her baby was "possessed" by evil spirits.)

GENERAL SCREENING QUESTIONS

BIRTH

How old are you?	*¿Cuántos años tiene usted?*
How many babies do you have?	*¿Cuántos niños tiene usted?*
How many months duration was your pregnancy?	*¿Cuánto meses duro su embarazo?*
How many days did you stay in the hospital?	*¿Cuántos días estuvo usted en el hospital?*
How many days did baby stay in the hospital?	*¿Cuántos días estuvo el niño en el hospital?*
What was baby's birth weight (pounds & ounces)?	*¿Cuánto peso el niño al nacer (libras y onzas)?*

CONSTITUTIONAL

Does your baby have any...?	*¿Tiene su niño algunas...?*
...Fevers/Chills	*...Fiebres/Escalofríos*
...Cough/Vomiting	*...Tosiendo/Vomitando*
...Runny Nose	*...Catarro (En La Nariz)/Moquean*
...Diarrhea/Constipation	*...Diarrea/Estreñimiento*
...Jaundice Or Yellow Skin	*...Icterica O La Piel Amarilla*
...Ear Infections	*...Infecciones De Las Orejas*
...Gastroenteritis	*...Gastroenteritis*
...Convulsions (with/without fever)	*...Convulsiones (con/sin fiebre)*
...Crying	*...Llorigueo (ó llanto)*
...Eye discharge	*...Desecho de los ojos*
...Unusual Stools	*...Escrementos inusuales*
Stools - Hard or Soft?	*Pupú/Las Haces - ¿Duro o suave?*
Loose or watery?	*¿Suelto o aguado?*
Of what color?	*¿De qué color?*
Is there changes with baby since the baby was last seen here (by the doctor)?	*¿Hay algunos cambios con el bebé desde la última vez eve vío (al doctor) aquí?*

FEEDS

Baby takes the breasts or the bottle?	*¿Toma el niño la botella o el pecho?*
How many minutes each breast/side?	*¿Cuántos minutos cada pecho/lado?*
What kind of formula?	*¿Qué clase de formula?*
How many ounces?	*¿Cuántas onzas?*
How many times a day?	*¿Cuántas veces al días?*
Don't feed the baby when he/she is laying...	*No le de comer al bebé cuando este acostado...*
Don't feed the baby while he/she is laying down...	*No alimente a su niño mientras que esta acostado boca arriba...*
Milk can penetrate into the ears and cause an infection...	*Leche puede penetrar en los oídos y causarle una infection...*
Milk can go to the ears and cause an infection...	*Leche puede ir a los oídos y causar una infection...*
Does baby take vitamins, fluoride, iron?	*¿El niño toma vitaminas, fluoruro, hierro?*
What do you feed your baby?	*Que le da de comer a su bebé?*
...formula (only)	*...formula (únicamente)*
...milk (only)	*...leche (únicamente)*
...solid foods	*...comida solidas*
...baby food from jars (eats gerber), bottles, cans	*...comida de frasco (comer gerber), botellas, botes.*
Your baby needs to take vitamins, iron, fluoride	*Su bebé necesita tomar vitaminas, hierro, floruro*

SLEEP

Are you getting enough rest?	*¿Está usted recibiendo suficiente reposo (ó decanso)?*
Does your baby sleep all the night?	*¿Su bebé duerme toda la noche?*
Does your baby sleep during the night? All night?	*Su bebé duerme durante la noche? Todo le noche?*
For how many hours does baby sleep at night?	*¿Por cuantas horas el bebé duerme en la noche?*
How many hours do you sleep each night?	*¿Cuantas horas usted duerme cada noche?*
How many hours does baby sleep each night?	*¿Cuantas horas el bebé duerme cada noche?*
Your baby/Your baby is...	*Su bebé/Su bebé está...*

...Sleep all the time	*...duerme todo el tiempo*
...Hard to wake up	*...difícil de despertarlo*
...Not sleeping well	*...No está durmiendo bien*
...Not sleep for the entire night	*...no duerme por todo la noche*

SAFETY

Do you have a car seat for the baby?	*¿Tiene asiento de seguridad para el niño?*
You have to get one... it's the law!	*¡Tiene que tener uno... es la ley!*
Do you have a smoke alarm in your house?	*¿Tiene alarma para incendio en su casa?*

HOME

Any persons sick at your home?	*¿Alguna persona está enferma en su casa?*
Are things going well at home?	*¿Las cosas van bien en la casa?*
Are your other children healthy? Any diarrhea, constipation, or fevers?	*¿Sus otros hijos, estan saludables? ¿Alguna diarrea, estreñmiento, ó fiebre?*
Do you have someone (a friend or relative) to help (to talk to) when things are difficult?	*¿Usted tiene alguien como (amigo-a ó un pariente) que le ayude (que pueda hablar) cuando las cosas se ponen dificultosas?*
Do you work? Are you going to work?	*¿Usted trabaja? ¿Usted está viendo a trabajar?*
Have you been feeling depressed after you had the baby?	*¿Se ha sentido deprimida después de tener el niño?*
The father (of the baby) lives with you?	*¿El Papa (de su bebé) vive con usted?*
Have you had any unexpected tragedy or severe stress (worry) in the family since your last visit?	*¿A tenido alguna trajedía inexperada ó bastante extrecha-miento (preoccupación) en su familia desde la ultima visita?*
How many adults live in your house?	*¿Cuántos personas adultas viven en su casa?*
How many children live in your house?	*¿Cuántos niños viven en su casa?*
Your husband helps with the baby?	*¿Le ayuda su esposo con el ninõ?*

Your husband/wife helps with the baby?	*¿Su esposo/esposa ayuda con el bebé?*

VACCINATIONS/ALLERGY

Do you have a dog or cat?	*Tiene una perro ó gato?*
Do you have your (blue), (green), (red), (yellow) card?	*¿Tiene su tarjeta (azul), (verde), (roja), (amarilla)?*
Does your family suffer from allergies?	*¿Padece/Sufre su familia de alérgias?*
Is your baby allergic to any medicines or foods?	*¿Es su niño alergico a alguna medicina o comida?*
One vaccination is an injection (shot). One vaccination is drops for the mouth.	*Una vacuna es una inyección. Una vacunaes una esta gotas por la boca.*
Your baby needs a (some) vaccination(s)	*Su bebé necesita (algunas) vacunas*

PERSONALITY

Can you tell me (in one word) the personality of your baby?	*Me puede decir (en una palabra) la personalidad de su bebé?*
Your baby/Your baby is...	*Su bebé/Su bebé está...*
...Happy/Sad	*...Feliz/Triste*
...Cry all the time	*...llora todo el tiempo*
...Cry easily	*...llora facilmente*
...Fussy	*...Fastidioso*
...Good/Bad	*...Bueno/Malo*
...Perfect	*...Perfecto*
...Rotten	*...Podridó*
...Spoiled	*...Concentido/Chipil*
...Unpredictable	*...Inesperado*
Are you content to have the baby?	*Está usted contenta de tener a su bebé?*
Are you worried about spoiling your baby?	*Se preocupa por concentir a su bebé?*

NEWBORN SCREENING

Do you have a thermometer?	*¿Tiene una termometro?*
Can you take the temperature of your baby?	*¿Puede usted tomar la temperatura del niño?*
Show me how...	*Enséñeme/Muestreme como...*
How many times a day do you clean the umbilical cord?	*¿Cuántos veces al día usted limpia el ombiligo?*
You have to clean the umbilicus 4-5 times a day	*Usted tiene que limpiar el ombligo cuatro-cinco veces al dia...*
The blood tests of your baby are normal/abnormal...	*Las pruebas de sangre de su niño son normales/ anormales...*
Is there anything you would like to ask the Doctor?	*¿Hay algo más qué usted quiere preguntarle al doctor/médico?*

Any problems with...	*Algunos problemas con...*
...Feeding	*...Alimentación*
...Crying	*...Lloriqueo (ó llanto)*
...Unusual Stools	*...Escrementos inusuales*
...Umbilical (cord) cleaning	*...Limpiezá (del cordón) ombilical*
...Eye discharge	*...Desecho de los ojos*
...Not eat enough/Eat too much	*...no comé lo suficiente, comé demasiado*
Does baby hear well?	*El bebé escucha bien?*
The baby turns to look when he hears loud noise?	*El bebé voltea a ver, cuando escucha sonidos fuertes?*

Do you know why baby cries (when he does cry)?	*Sabe usted por que se bebé llora (cuando el llorá)?*
...Hungry	*...hambre*
...Tired	*...cansancio*
...Cold	*...Fríos (Calofrios)*
...Too much activity	*...demasiada (ó mucha) actividad*
...Too much noise	*...muchos ruidos*
...Uncomfortable	*...inconfortable*
...Belly pain	*...dolor de estomago*
...Ear Pain	*...dolor de oído*

Pulling on the ears?	*¿Se jala las orejas?*

DEVELOPMENTAL MILESTONES

FINE MOTOR

Hands together	*Junta las manos*
Eye/Head follows object	*Los Ojos/Cabeza sigue objectos*
Looks at raisin	*Mira a la paza*
Grasps rattle	*Agara el jugete*
Sits, looks for yarn	*Acentado lo busca*
Picks up Cheerios (cereals)	*Recoje los Cheerios (Cereales)*
Sribbles with crayons	*Debuja/Garrapatos con lapiz de color*
Write the letter "O"	*Escribe la letra "O"*
Writes "+"	*Escribe "+"*
Writes "□"	*Escribe "□"*
Draws stick figure man	*Debeja un hombre de palitos*

LANGUAGE

Laughs	*Reir (Se rie)*
Squeals	*Chillido/Soplón*
Vocalizes (Not Crying)	*Vocaliza (Sin Llorar)*
Turns to voice	*Voltea a la voz*
Says "Mama" & "Dada"	*Dice "Mama" & "Papa"*
Sentence of 3 words	*Frase de tres palabras*
Gives first name	*Da su nombre (primero)*
Gives last name	*Da su apellido*
Knows hot from cold	*Conoce caliente de frio*
Knows orange from red	*Conoce anaranjado de colorado*
Knows green from blue	*Conoce verde de azul*

GROSS MOTOR

Lifts head	*Levanta la cabeza*
Rolls over	*Se voltea a bocariba*
Sits With Support	*Se Sienta Con Soporte*
Sits without support	*Se sienta sin apollo/sin soporte*
Stands holding on	*Se para agarado*
Pulls self to stand	*Se para solo*
Can Stay On Feet With Support	*Se Mantiene De Pie Soportándose*

Gets to sitting without help	*Se sienta solo*
Walks holding onto furniture	*Camina cuando se agara de los muebles*
Stoops to pick up object	*se agacha para recojer cosas*
Walks backwards	*Camina alrevez*
Walks up steps	*Sube Escalones*
Kicks ball	*Patalea pelotas*
Throws the ball	*Tira la pelota*
Jumps in place	*Brinca en un lugar*
Balances on (1) foot	*Se balance en un pie*
Hops on (1) foot	*Brinca en un pie*

PERSONAL

Smiles	*Sonria*
Smiles At Mom (Spontaneously)	*Sonrisas A La Mamá (Espontáneamente)*
Feeds self	*Come solo/Se Alimenta*
Resists pull	*Resiste cuando lo jala*
Shy with strangers	*Tiene miedo de desconocidos*
Plays ball	*Juega pelota*
Drinks from cup	*Toma de tasa*
Imitates work	*Imita trabajo*
Removes clothes alone	*Se quita la ropa solo*
Uses spoon	*Usa la quchara*
Helps in house	*Ayuda en casa*
Puts on clothes	*Se pone la ropa/Se viste*
Wash/Dry hands	*Se lava/Seca las manos*
Plays games with others	*Juega juegos con otros*
Dresses with help	*Se viste con ayuda*

Return with your baby if...	*Regrese con el niño si...*

Please bring/return the baby to this clinic (or emergency) if he has...	*Por favor traiga/regrese al niño de regreso a esta clinica o a emergencia si tiene...*
...Fever (above 102°F)	*...Fiebre (arriba de 102°F)*
...Diarrhea for 3 days	*...Diarrhea por tres (3) días*
...Vomiting	*...Vomitos*
...Not eating	*...No come/Sin comer*
...Problems breathing	*...Problemas al respirar*
...Problems with waking your baby	*...Problemas para despiertarlo su niño*
...Sleeping too much	*...Durmiendo demaciado*
Come back when baby is __ weeks/months old.	*Regresé cuando el bebé es __ semanas/meses de edad.*

ODD TOPICS

- SPANISH PRONUNCIATION/ALPHABET
- PHLEBOTOMY (BLOOD DRAWING)
- ANESTHESIA/PRE-OP EVALUATION
- POST-OP RECOMMENDATIONS
- DENTAL PHRASES
- PRESCRIPTION ORDERS

SPANISH PRONUNCIATION

The Latinic pronunciation of the 5 vowels differs from English.
Also, the Latinic alphabet contains several consonants not found
in the English alphabet.

Vowel	Name	Spanish Sound
A	A	"AH" as in "Blah" or "On Call"
E	E	"A" as in "Late Night", "EH" as in "Fred" when after a consonant or at the beginning of a sentence
I	I	"EE" as in "Peek"
O	O	"O" as in "Got to go" when the last letter of a syllable.
U	U	"OO" as in "Loon", "W" when followed/preceded by another vowel, Silent in the combinations (GUE), (GUI), (QUE), & (QUI).

Consnts	Name	Spanish Sound
B	Be	"B" as in "Baseball" when at the beginning of a sentence or preceded by the letter (M). Now this is where it really gets strange, when between two vowels or between a vowel and the letters (L) or (R), then pronounced as "V"
C	Ce	"SS" as in "Bliss" or "K" when before a, o, or u.
Ch	Che	"CH" as is "what's up Chuck?"
D	De	"D" as in "Dog" or as "TH" as in "There" when between two vowels or followed by the letter (R).
F	Efe	"F" as in "Fluoride Tooth Paste"
G	Ge	"H" as in "Home Run!" when before an (E) or (I). "G" as in "Get Smart!" when before an (A), (O), or (U).
H	Hache	Silent "Hola!" becomes "Ola!"
J	Jota	"H" as in "Hard work, Jose"
L	Ele	"L" as in "Lousy Cafeteria Food"
Ll	Elle	"Y" as in "Yankee", "Tortillas" becomes "Torti-yas."
M	Eme	"M" as in "Mutant Samari Lizards™"
N	Ene	"N" as in "New York", "M" when before a (V), or "N" as in "Think" when before (C) or (G).
Ñ	Eñe	"NY" as in "Nyuk-Nyuk-Nyuk" or "Canyon"
P	Pe	"P" as in "Please Urinate" though it can be silent in Spanish as in "séptimo"
Q	Cu	"K" as in "Kind Hearted"
R	Ere	Trilled "R" when after an (L), (N), or (S). Otherwise, "R" as in "Run Spot Run!"
Rr	Erre	Trilled "R" as in "R-R-Rolling R-R-Rapids"
S	Ese	"SS" as in "Bliss"
T	Te	"T" as in "Tiempo (time)"
V	Ve	"B" as in "Scuba"
X	Equis	"S" when followed by a consonant, "GS" as in "Eggs" when between two vowels.
Y	Ye	"I" in "machine" or "Y" when following a vowel.
Z	Zeda	"SS" as in "Bliss"
K or W		Not found in Spanish words (few rare exceptions)

Diphthong	Spanish Sound
ia	"yuh" as is "Mala<u>ria</u>"
ie	"ee-ye" (diente (tooth) = d<u>ee</u>-<u>ye</u>n-tay)
io	"ee-yo" as in Rad<u>io</u>
iu	"you" as in "Hey <u>you</u> dumb jerk"
ua	"wuh" as in "<u>Wuh</u> did you say?"
ue	"weh" as in "Nice <u>wea</u>ther we're having!"

The only way you are going to learn the pronunciation is by
 (1) *Listening to your patients*
 (2) *Trying to reproduce the words you hear*

The only way you are going to learn the vocabulary is by
 (1) *Having a friend ask you the word/phrase in English and you give the Spanish equivalent*
 (2) *Practicing the vocabulary with your patients and seeing that it really does work.*

PHLEBOTOMY (BLOOD DRAWING)

Hello, my name is Doctor ...	¡Hola! Me llamo Doctor ...
Dr. Dracula/Vampire (small bit of humor)	Dr. Dracúla/Vampiro ...
Don't be afraid...	No tenga miedo...
I need to take a sample of blood...	Necesito sacar una meustra de sangre ...
I need to start an I.V....	Necesito empazarle un suero...
I need [7] tubes...	Necesito [siete] tubos...
Lift up your sleeve...	Súbase la manga...
Extend your arm...	Extienda el brazo...
Straighten the arm please...	El brazo mas recto, por favor...
Close/Open your hand...	Cierra/Abra la mano...
Relax/Rest your arm...	Relajese/Descanse el brazo ...
Move your fingers...	Meuve los dedos...
Make a fist...	Haga un puño...
You will feel a little stick...	Va a sentir un piquitito/pica .
Don't move please...	No se mueva por favor...
I could not obtain enough blood...	No pude obtener bastante sangre...
Another stick...	Otro pica/piquitito...
I'm sorry... another time...	Lo siento... otra vez...
Are you dizzy?	¿Está mareado?
Put your head between the legs...	Pongo la cabeza en medio las piernas...
Press here to stop the bleeding...	Apriete aquí para parar la sangre...
I will return in one and a half hours...	Regresaré en una hora y media...

ANESTHESIA & PRE-OP EVALUATION

I am going to give you anesthesia (tomorrow)	*Yo le daré la anestesia (mañana)*
An associate is going to give the anesthesia	*Algún asociado le va a dar el anestético*
What is your name?	*¿Cómo se llama?*
How many years do you have (age)?	*¿Cuántos años tienes (edad)?*
How much do you weigh (in pounds)?	*¿Cuanto pesa (en libras)?*
Height "stature" (in feet)?	*¿Estatura (en pies)?*
Date of the operation?	*¿Fecha de la operación?*
Name of the operation?	*¿Nombre de la operación?*
What kind of surgery are you going to have?	*¿Que clase de cirugía ira tener?*
Have you ever had surgery before?	*¿Ha tenido algunas operaciones antes?*
Did you have problems with the anesthesia?	*¿Tuvo algún problems con la anestesia?*
Were you awake or asleep?	*¿Estuvo desperto o dormido?*
You are going to have...	*Usted ira tener...*
...General anesthesia (for all the body)	*...Anestesia general (para todo el cuerpo)*
...Local anesthesia (for part of the body)	*...Anestesia local (para parte el cuerpo)*
...You will be asleep/awake	*...Usted estará durmiendo/ despiertado*
Do you take medicines?	*¿Toma usted medicina?*
Have problems taking medicines?	*¿Tiene problemas al tomar medicinas?*
Do you have any allergies?	*¿Tiene alergias?*
Has anyone in your family had...?	*¿Hay alguien en su familia haya tenido...?*
...Problems with anesthesia?	*...Problemas con anestesia?*
...A bleeding tendency?	*...Tendencia a sangrar?*
Have you had an illness in the last two weeks?	*¿Ha estado enfermo en las últimas dos semanas?*

Smoke?	*¿Fuma?*
How many packs a day?	*¿Cuántos paquetes al días?*
Drink?	*¿Toma/beba?*
How much a day?	*¿Cuántos a días?*
For how many years?	*¿Por cuántos años?*
Use drugs?	*¿Usa drogas?*
Do you have high blood pressure?	*¿Tiene alta presión?*
Do you have problems breathing at night?	*¿Tiene problemas al respirar a noche?*
Do you have any heart disease?	*¿Tiene algunas enfermedad del corazón?*
Do you have any bleeding tendency?	*¿Tiene algunas tendencia a sangrar?*
Do you have problems with your liver? Cirrhosis? Hepatitis?	*¿Tiene problemas con su hígado? ¿Cirrosis? ¿Hepatitis?*
Do you have a need for steroids?	*¿Tiene necesidad de esteroides?*

Do you have problems opening your mouth/jaw (mandible)?	*¿Tiene problemas para abrir la boca/quijada (mandíbula)?*
Do you have problems moving the jaw (mandible) or the neck?	*¿Tiene problemas para mover la quijada (mandíbula) o el cuello?*
Do you have loose teeth?	*¿Tiene dientes flojos/sueltos?*
Do you have loose crowns?	*¿Tiene coronas flojos/sueltos?*
Do you have broken teeth?	*¿Tiene dientes astillados?*
Do you have contact lenses?	*¿Tiene lentes de contacto?*
Do you have a hearing aid?	*¿Tiene una audíofono?*

Have you had breakfast?	*¿Tomó desayuno?*
Have you eaten since midnight?	*¿Ha comido desde la medianoche?*
When was your last meal? Before midnight?	*¿Cuándo fue la última vez que comió? ¿Antes de medianoche?*
Don't eat/drink after midnight...	*No comé/bebé después de medianoche...*
Nothing by mouth...	*Nada por la boca...*

Except for your medicines...	*Aparte de sus medicinas...*

This is the... Operating Room/Recovery Room...	*Esta es la sala de operación/ sala de recuperación...*
Move here... to the middle of this bed...	*Muevase aquí... al medio de este cama...*
Breath with this mask...	*Respire con esta mascara...*
It is (only) oxygen...	*Esto es (solamente) oxigeno...*
Wake up! Open your eyes!	*¡Desperta! ¡Abra sus ojos!*
Your surgery is complete!	*¡Se acabó la cirugía!*
Everything went well...	*Todo salió bien...*

POST-OP RECOMMENDATIONS

DIET	DIETA
Begin with a diet of clear liquids...	Empiece con una dieta de líquidos claros...
Begin with a light diet...	Empiece con una dieta ligera...
Don't take hot liquids for two days...	No tome liquidos calientes por dos dias...
Follow with other foods as you can tolerate...	Siga con otros alimentos/ comidas según los vaya tolerando...
Take plenty of liquids...	Tome bastante líquidos...
When you recover your appetite...	Cuando recobre el apetito...
You can take clear liquids when awake and alert...	Puede tomar líquidos claros cuando despierte y altera...
...clear liquids	...líquidos claro
...bland foods	...comidas blandas
...puréed foods	...comidas hechas puré

ACTIVATIES	ACTIVIDAD
Avoid hitting at the site of incision...	Evite pegarse en el lugar de la incisión...
Do not exercise...	No haga ejercicios...
Don't blow your nose...	No se suene la nariz...
Elevate the arm/leg...	Eleve/Levante el brazo/la pierna...
Elevate the head of the bed...	Levante la cabecera de la cama...
If you need to sneeze, do so with the mouth open...	Si necesita estornudar, hágalo con la boca abierta...
No/Avoid heavy lifting...	No levante/Evite levantar cosas pesadas...
Put no pressure over the site where you had the fracture repaired...	No se ponga presion sobre el lugar donde le han reparado la fractura...
Rest today, later you can resume your normal activities...	Descanse hoy, después puede reanudar sus actividades normales...
Sit in warm water and allow for 10-15 minutes four times a day (after defecating)...	Siéntese en agua caliente según la consienta por 10-15 minutos cuatro veces al día (después de defecar)...

Stay in bed the day of the operation (except when you have to go to the bathroom)...	Quedace/Permenezca en cama el día de la operación (excepto cuando tenga que ir al baño)...
Tomorrow you can resume your activities if you feel in condition...	Mañana puede reanudar sus actividades si se siente en condiciones...
Use pillows during the night to keep the head elevated...	Usa almohadas durante la noche para mantener la cabeza elevada...
You can climb stairs...	Puede subir escaleras...
You can drive a car...	Puede pasear en coche...
You can not put weight on the leg...	No se permite poner peso en la pierna...
You can put complete weight on the leg...	Se permite poner peso completo en la pierna...
You can put moderate weight on the leg...	Se permite poner peso moderado en la pierna...
You can take a shower or bath...	Puede darse baños de duche o tina...
You can walk...	Puede caminar...
You should not have (sexual) relations if you feel discomfort	No debe tener relaciones (sexuales) si siente molestias

CONSIDERATIONS

CONSIDERACIONES

Don't worry if you can't hear well during the first ___ weeks...	No se preocupe si no puede oír bien durante las primeras ___ semanas
It is normal to have moderate pain after the operation...	Es normal tener dolor moderado depués de la operación...
It is possible that you have abominal pain and/or pain in the shoulders...	Es posible que usted tenga el abdomen adolorido y/o dolor en los hombros...
It is possible to have discomfort at defecating after the operation...	Es posible que tenga molestias para defecar después de la operación...
The urine will have a light tint of blood and small clots during the first 24 hours...	La orina tendrá un ligero tinte de sangre y pequeños coágulos durante las primeras vientecuatro horas...

WOUND CARE/ DRESSING
CUIDAD DE LA HERIDA / VENDAJE

Avoid putting adhesive tape & guaze around the arm or the leg...	*Evite ponerse cinta adhesiva y gasa alrededor del brazo o pierna...*
Change the bandage when it is saturated with blood...	*Cámbiese el vendaje cuando esté saturado de sange...*
Change the bandage...	*Cámbiese el vendaje...*
Continue to use sanitary napkins to retain the blood...	*Continúe usando toallas sanitarias para retener la sangre...*
Do not put on (tight) fitting cloths...	*No se ponga ropa ajustada...*
Don't remove the bandage...	*No se quite el vendaje...*
If you have "Steri-Strips" on the incision, leave them until they peel off themselves...	*Si le ponen "Steri-Strips" sobre la incisión, déjeselas hasta que se le caigan solas...*
Keep the ears dry...	*Mantenga los oídos secos*
Keep the site of the incision covered with a sterile and dry bandage...	*Mantenga el lugar de la incisión cubierto con un vendaje estéril y seco...*
The bandages can be removed the day of the operation...	*Los vendajes pueden quitarse el día después de la operación...*
You can shower or take a bath, but don't scrub the site of the incision...	*Puede ducharse o darse un baño de tina, pero no se restregue el lugar de la incisión...*

MEDICINES FOR PAIN
MEDICINAS PARA DOLOR

Take the medicine prescribed by the doctor...	*Tome la medicina recetada por el médico/doctor...*

APPOINTMENT
CITA

Ear, Nose, and Throat Clinic	*Clínica de Oídos, Nariz, y Garganta*
General Surgery Clinic	*Clínica de Cirugía General*
GYN Clinic	*Clínica de Ginecología*
Orthopedic Clinic	*Clínica de Ortopedia*
Urology Clinic	*Clínica de Urologia*

EMERGENCY ROOM
SALA DE EMERGENCIAS

Go to our Emergency Room (or call the doctor) if...	*Venga a nuestra sala de emergencias (o llame al médico) si...*

If a lot of blood by rectum...	*Si sangra mucho del recto...*
If the pain worsens...	*Si le empeora el dolor...*
If you feel numbness, tingling, or severe throbbing pain...	*Si siente adormecimiento, hormigueo, o dolor pulante muy fuertes...*
If you have any problems breathing...	*Si tiene dificultad para respirar...*
If you have chills or fever over (101°F)...	*Si tiene escalofríos o fiebre de más de 101°F...*
If you have discharge of blood vaginally (which is more than your normal period)...	*Si tiene flujo de sangre vaginal (cual es más abundante que su regla normal)...*
If you have discharge with bad smell...	*Si tiene flujo con mal olor...*
If you have excessive bleeding at the site of the incision...	*Si tiene sangra excesivamente el lugar de la incisión...*
If you have not passed gas (by rectum) 24 hours after the operation...	*Si no ha podido pasar gas (por el recto) vienticuatro horas después de la operación...*
If you have pain in the chest or the back...	*Si tiene dolor en el pecho o en la espalda...*
If you have pus...	*Si le sale pus...*
If you have redness around the wound...	*Si tiene enrojecimiento alrededor de la herida...*
If you have severe cramps...	*Si tiene calambres fuertes...*
If you have swelling or sufficient pain...	*Si tiene muy hinchado o bastante dolor...*
If you have warmth/pain/ swelling/redness at the site of the incision...	*Si tiene caliente /le duele / hinchada /enrojecimiento a lugar de la incisión...*
If you have whatever sign of infection...	*Si tiene cualquier síntoma de infección...*
The bandage becomes saturated with blood...	*El vendaje se satura de sangre...*
The urine had a lot of blood (the color clear red) or large clots...	*La orina mucha sangre (de color rojo claro) o coágulos grandes...*
You cannot urinate for a period greater than 8 hours after the operation...	*No puede orinar por un período de más de ocho horas después de su operación...*

DENTAL

abscess	absceso	full denture	dentadura completa
baby teeth	dientes de leche	gum infection	infeccion de las encias
bicuspid	bicuspide	inflamed gums	encias inflamadas
bridge	puente	root	raiz
cavity	carie	saliva	saliva
cleaning	limpieza	tongue	lengua
crown	corona	toothache; back	dolor de muelas
decayed tooth	diente cariado	toothache; front	dolor de dientes
dental clinic	clinica dental	toothbrush	cepillo de dientes
drill	taladro	treatments	tratamientos
extraction	extraccion		
impacted wis-dom tooth	muela del juicio impactado	roof of the mouth	cielo de la boca

bleed (v.)	sangrar	drill (v.)	taladrar
brush teeth (v.)	cepillar los dientes	extract (v.)	extraer
chew (v.)	masticar	fill (v.)	empastar
clean the teeth (v.)	limpiar los dientes	rinse (v.)	enjuagarse
deaden the nerve (v.)	adormecer el nervio		
spit in the cup (v.)	escupir en la taza		

How long since you visited a dentist?
¿Cuanto tiempo hace que no visita una dentista?

Does it hurt when you drink something hot or cold?
Le duele cuando toma algo caliente ó frio?

Point to where it hurts
Apunte donde le duele

Open your mouth
Abra la boca

Open wider
Abrala más

This tooth?
¿Este diente?

It's impacted
Está impactada

I have to extract it
Yo tango que extraerla

You have...
Usted tiene ...

...(__) cavities (caries)
...(__) caries.

...an abscess
...una absceso

...a decayed tooth
...un diente cariado

...a gum infection
...un infeccion de las encias

...lost a filling	...*perdido un empaste/relleno*
Your teeth need to be cleaned	*Sus dientes necesitan una limpieza*
What kind of filling do you want?	*Qué clase de relleno quiere?*
...**gold**	...*oro*
...**porcelain**	...*porcelana*
...**silver**	...*plata*
You need...	*Necesita...*
...**a bridge**	...*un puente*
...**a crown (to cover the tooth)**	...*una corona (para cubrir el diente)*
...**a filling**	...*un empaste/relleno*
...**a full denture**	...*una dentadura completa*
...**a partial denture**	...*una dentadura parcial*
...**a toothbrush**	...*un cepillo de dientes*
...**treatments**	...*tratamientos*
I am going to give you an injection of anesthetic	*Le voy a darle una inyección de anestético*
Spit in the cup	*Escupa en la taza*

Spanish Note: Two words are commonly used for a dental filling ("*un empaste*" and "*un relleno*"). You'll just have to try both and see which word works best. You may recognize the second word, "*relleno*," from the popular Mexican dish, *chilé relleno*, which means "chilé filling."

PRESCRIPTION ORDERS

Medicine	*Medicinas*	Drops	*Gotas*
Prescription	*Receta*	Syrup	*Jarabe*
Pills	*Píldoras*	Ointment	*Pomada*
Tablets	*Pastillas/ Tableta*	Lozenge	*Oblea*

INSTRUCTIONS

Eat this	*Coma esto*	Soak this	*Remojar esto*
Drink this	*Beba esto*	Rub this	*Frotar esto*
Swallow this	*Trague esto*	Bring this	*Traiga esto*
Chew this	*Mastique esto*	Hold this	*Agarre esto*
Inhale this	*Inhalar esto*	Keep this	*Mantenga esto*
Apply this	*Aplicar esto*	Swallow it	*Tráguela*

Take this medicine	*Tome esta medicina*
Take this (ingest this)	*Tome esto*
Don't swallow it	*No la trague*
Don't chew it	*No la mastique*
Take (__) pills/tablets	*Tome (__) pildoras/pastillas*
By mouth (po)	*Por la boca*
By rectum (pr)	*En el recto*
One a day (qd)	*Una vez por día*
Twice a day (bid)	*Dos veces por día*
Three times a day (tid)	*Tres veces al día*
Four times a day (qid)	*Cuatro veces al día*
Every other day (qod)	*Cada otra día*
Every (__) hours (q __ hrs)	*Cada (__) horas*
Before meals (ac)	*Antes de las comidas*
After meals (pc)	*Después de las comidas*
With meals	*Con las comidas*
Between meals	*Entre comidas*
Before going to bed (qhs)	*Antes de acostarse*
When you get up in the morning (qAM)	*Cuando se levante por la mañana*
When necessary	*Cuando necesario*
Every day	*Todos los día*
Each day	*Cada día*
For (__) days	*Por (__) días*
For the rest of your life	*Por todo la vida*
Take this with food	*Tome esto con comida*
Take this on an empty stomach	*Tome esto con estómago vacío*
You have to finish all of the medicine	*Usted tiene que terminar toda la medicina*
Bring me the bottles and medicines	*Tráigame las botellas y medicinas*

LISTS - PHRASES

- **COMMON FIRST PHRASES**
- **GREETINGS & SALUTATIONS**
- **COMFORTING PHRASES**
- **GENERAL PURPOSE MEDICAL PHRASES**
- **COMMON POLICE PHRASES**

COMMON FIRST PHRASES

FIRST LINES

I am just learning to speak Spanish...	*Yo estoy apenas aprendiendo a hablar Español...*
I don't speak good Spanish...	*No hablo muy bien español...*
I'm reading from a list of questions...	*Estoy leyendo de un questionario varias preguntas...*
That I need to know about you...	*Que necesito saber de usted...*
Please answer "yes" or "no" to my questions...	*Por favor conteste "si" o "no" a mis preguntas...*
Please answer my questions slowly...	*Por favor conteste mis preguntas despacio...*
Write down the number...	*Escriba el numero...*
Write down the date...	*Escriba la fecha...*
Speak slowly...	*Hable despacio...*
Can you speak more slowly?	*¿Puedes hablar más despacio?*
Not so fast!	*¡No tan rápido!*
I don't know...	*No sé...*
I dunno...	*No sabé...*
I don't get it...	*Me no sabé...*
I don't understand...	*No entiendo...*
Do you understand?	*¿Entiende usted?*
Pardon me, What did you say?	*¿Mande?*
You tell me and we'll both know...	*Usted digame y los dos llegaremos a saber...*
In what way can I help you?	*¿En que le puedo ayudar?*

Cultural Note: Many of my Mexican patients are fatalistic and very fond of sayings. The proverb, "Todo ira bien...¡Si Dios es servido!" ("All will go well... if God is served") works very well to relieve anxiety while, "Con paciencia se gana el cielo" ("With patience, one can gain heaven") works very well to relieve frustration. It is terribly important that you do not confuse "pena" (pains) with "pene" (penis). "Me da pena" changes it's meaning otherwise.

GREETINGS/SALUTATIONS

Hello/Goodbye	!Hola¡/¡Adiós!
Good day/afternoon	Buenos dias/tardes
Good evening/night	Buenas noches
My name is...	Me llamo...
Sir, Madam, Miss	Señor, Señora, Señorita
Dr. ____, at your service!	Doctor ____, ¡a sus órdenes!
Welcome	¡Bienvenido!
Until Later/Until I see you...	Hasta Luego/Hasta la vista
Please (beginning of a sentence)	Favor de...
Please (end of a sentence)	...por favor.
How are you?	¿Cómo está usted?
Thank you very much	Muchas gracias
Excuse me ("with your permission")	Con su permiso
Pardon me.	Perdón
It's a pleasure.	Mucho gusto
Until the next visit.	Hasta la próxima cita
Thanks "of nothing"	De Nada
Thanks "don't mention it"	No hay de qué
Very Good/Well	Muy Bien
Congradulations	Felicidades
Good Luck.	¡Buena suerte!
How do you say __ in Spanish?	¿Cómo se dice __ en español?

Cultural Note: "¿Mande? ¿Mande?" literally "How How?" is an idiom from Mexico originally used when speaking to royalty roughly meaning, "what is thy command?" Today it can be translated for, "excuse me, what did you say?" Repeating this again and again will inform the patient that you don't speak Spanish in a more convincing way of saying "I don't understand (No entiendo)."

COMFORTING PHRASES

After - to your home!	*Después - ¡a la casa!*
All will go well...	*Todo ira bien...*
At your service...	*A sus órdenes...*
Calm down (dude) ...	*Cálmese (amigo)...*
Don't complain so much...	*No se queje tanto...*
Don't worry (you rat) ...	*No se preocupe (ratón) ...*
Have to operate...	*Hay que operar...*
How are you?	*¿Coma está?*
How is my favorite patient?	*¿Como está mi paciente predilecta?*
How is my Mexican friend?	*¿Como está mi amigo Mexicano?*
I'll give you an enema...	*Le daré una enema...*
I'm sorry... ("it pains me")	*Me da pena...*
If God wills ... ("is served")	*Si Dios es servido...*
It pains me... to your home today!	*Me da pena...¡A la casa hoy!*
It was a pleasure to work with you...	*Fué un placer el hacer este trabajo...*
It was a pleasure treating you...	*Fué un placer tratarle...*
Some days in the hospital!	*¡Unos días en el hospital!*
Take a chill pill...	*Tome un resfrío pildora...*
Thanks for everything...	*Gracias por todo...*
There is no cancer...	*No hay cáncer ...*
Very glad to have served you...	*Muy contento en haberle servido...*
We all do the best we can...	*Todo nosotros hace mos le mejor que podemos...*
What a pity...	*Qué lástima...*
What's the matter?	*¿Qué le pasa?*
With patience, one can gain heaven...	*Con paciencia se gana el cielo...*
You are cured...	*Usted está curado...*
You musn't be afraid!	*¡No hay que llorar!*
You are going to live...	*Usted va a vivir...*
You will not die...	*Usted no va a morir...*

GENERAL PURPOSE MEDICAL PHRASES

a.c.; before meals	*antes de las comidas*
a.m. "in the morning"	*de la mañana*
absolutely not	*absolutamente no*
after - to your home!	*después - ¡a la casa!*
after meals (p.c.)	*después de las comidas*
after tomorrow	*pasado mañana*
all will go well	*todo ira bien*
allow me to introduce myself	*permítame presentarme*
already!	*¡ya!*
am I speaking clearly	*hablo claramente*
are you coming with me?	*¿usted me acompaña?*
are you lost	*está perdido*
are you sure?	*¿estaseguro?*
are you thirsty?	*¿tiene sed?*
as for me	*en cuanto a mi*
at any rate anyway	*en todo caso*
at any time	*alguna vez*
at first	*al comienzo*
at home	*en casa*
at night (p.m.)	*de la noche*
at your service	*a sus órdenes*
be careful	*tenga cuidado*
before going to bed (q.hs)	*antes de acostarse*
before meals (a.c.)	*antes de las comidas*
better and better	*mejor y mejor*
better or worse	*mejor ó peor*
between meals	*entre comidas*
bring me the bottles and medicines	*traígame las botellas y medicinas*
bring this	*traiga esto*
by mouth (p.o.)	*por la boca*
by plane	*por avión*
by rectum (p.r.)	*en el recto*
by the way	*a propósito*
call this telephone number	*llame a este número de teléfono*
calm down (dude)	*cálmese (amigo)*
can I call you a taxi	*le llamo a un taxi*
can I have	*¿puedo tener?*
can you help me	*¿puedo ayudarme?*
can you prove this	*puede comprobar esto*
can you smell it?	*¿puede olerlo?*
can you speak more slowly?	*¿puedes hablar más despacio?*
can you speak slowly?	*¿puede hablar lento?*

can you tell me	¿puede decirme?
check this	revise esto
come closer	venga más cerca
come in	¡pase usted!
come tomorrow	venga mañana
congradulations	felicidades
consult with the specialist	consulte con el especialista
day by day	día a día
do like I tell you	haga como le digo
do you feel	se siente
do you have	tiene
do you know Mr. x	conoce usted al señor x
do you mean it?	¿en serio?
do you speak english?	¿habla usted inglés?
do you understand me?	¿me compriende usted?
do you understand?	¿entiende usted?
do you want it?	¿lo quiere?
doctor ____, at your service!	doctor ____, ¡a sus órdenes!
don't be afraid	no tenga miedo
don't complain so much	no se queje tanto
don't exaggerate	no exagere
don't move	no se mueva
don't pay any attention	no le haga caso
don't swallow it	no la trague
don't tell me that	no me diga eso
don't worry	no se preocupe
each day	cada día
eat this	coma esto
every day	todos los día
every other day (q.o.d)	cada otra día
excuse me ("with your permission")	con su permiso
fine, thanks, and you?	bien, gracias, ¿y usted?
follow the diet	siga la dieta
for (__) days	por (__) días
for rent	para alquilar
for the most part	la mayoría
for the rest of your life	por todo la vida
for what reason?	¿por dónde?
four times a day (q.i.d.)	cuatro veces al día
from now on	de ahora en adelante
from where?	¿de dónde?
get ready	prepárese
give me a hand	déme una mano

go straight ahead	*siga derecho*
good day/afternoon	*buenos dias/tardes*
good luck	*buena suerte*
good morning	*buenos días*
good night	*buenas noches*
good to have you back	*que bueno que esté de regreso*
goodbye	*adiós (used mainly by gringos)*
goodbye	*chau/chao/chaucito (used by natives)*
happy birthday	*feliz cumpleaños*
have a good trip	*tenga un buen viaje*
have to operate	*hay que operar*
have you had	*ha tenido*
have you noticed	*ha notado*
he is on his way	*está en camino*
hello	*!hola¡*
help	*ayuda*
help!	*¡socorro!*
here is	*aquí está*
hold this	*agarre esto*
how are you doing?	*¿cómo le va?*
how are you today?	*¿cómo está usted hoy?*
how are you?	*¿cómo está usted?, ¿qué tal?*
how can I help you?	*¿en qué puedo servirlo?*
how come?	*¿de cuándo acá?*
how do you feel	*cómo se siente*
how do you feel today?	*¿cómo se siente usted hoy?*
how do you say ___ in spanish?	*¿cómo se dice___ en español?*
how do you say ____?	*¿cómo se dice _____?*
how far?	*¿hasta dónde?*
how is my favorite patient?	*¿como está mi paciente predilecta?*
how is my Mexican friend?	*¿como está mi amigo Mexicano?*
how is your family?	*¿qué tal su familia?*
how long? (time)	*¿cuánto tiempo?*
how much do I owe	*cuánto le debo*
how much is it?	*¿cuánto es?*
how much is?	*¿a cómo es?*
how much?	*¿cuánto?*
how often do you ?	*¿qué tan seguido?*
how old are you?	*¿cuántos años tiene usted?*
how's everything?	*¿qué tal?*
how?	*¿cómo?*
hurry	*¡dése prisa!*
I am not sick	*yo no estoy enfermo*

I am not sore	*yo no estory enfadado*
I can do it	*lo puedo hacer*
I did it	*yo lo hice*
I did not do it	*yo no lo hice*
I did not see it	*yo no lo vi*
I didn't understand what I was doing	*yo no sabía lo que estaba haciendo*
I don't have time	*no tengo tiempo*
I don't know	*no sé*
I don't like it	*no me gusta*
I don't think so	*creo que no*
I don't understand	*no entiendo*
I feel better	*me siento mejor*
I found it	*lo encontré*
I knew it	*lo sabía*
I know him/her	*lo/la conozco*
I like ___	*me gusto __*
I need	*necisito*
I noticed that	*yo lo noté*
I see it	*lo veo*
I think so	*creo que sí*
I want	*Yo quiero*
I want a coffee, please	*Yo quiero un café por favor*
I want to speak with him	*Yo quiero hablar con él*
I was not a witness	*yo no fui testigo-a*
I was not there	*yo no estaba allí*
I will show you	*yo le enseñaré*
I won	*¡yo gané!*
I would like	*me gustaría*
I' m very sorry	*lo siento mucho*
I'll give you an enema	*le daré una enema*
I'll miss you	*le extrañaré*
I'm afraid	*tengo miedo*
I'm bored	*estoy aburrida*
I'm going to call the police!	*¡voy a llamar a la policia!*
I'm having a good time	*me estoy divirtiendo mucho*
I'm hungry	*tengo hambre*
I'm leaving	*me voy*
I'm sorry	*lo siento*
I'm sorry ("it pains me")	*me da pena*
I'm thirsty	*tengo sed*
I'm used to it	*estoy acostumbrado*
if God wills ("is served")	*si Dios es servido*

in front (straight ahead)	*adelante/derecho*
in the afternoon (p.m.)	*de la tarde*
in the morning (a.m.)	*de la mañana*
in what way can I help you?	*¿en que le puedo ayudar?*
inhale this	*inhalar esto*
is it far?	*¿esta lejos?*
is it open?	*¿está ablerto?*
it pains me to your home today!	*me da pena¡a la casa hoy!*
it smells good	*huele rico*
it started	*empezó*
it was a pleasure to work with you	*fué un placer el hacer este trabajo*
it was a pleasure treating you	*fué un placer tratarle*
it's a pleasure	*mucho gusto*
it's about time	*ya es tiempo*
it's all right	*está bien*
it's cold	*hace frio*
it's dirty	*está sucio*
it's easy	*es fácil*
it's good	*está bueno*
it's here	*está aquí*
it's hot	*hace calor*
it's my pleasure	*el piacer es para mi*
it's near here	*es cerca de aquí*
it's necessary	*es necesario*
it's nice weather	*hace buen tiempo*
it's not important	*no importa*
it's nothing	*no es nada*
it's obvious	*es obvio*
it's out of the question	*de ningun modo*
it's over	*se acabó*
it's the same	*yo mismo*
it's time to go	*es hora de irse*
it's too late	*es demasiado tarde*
it's true	*es verdad*
keep moving	*siga moviéndose*
keep the change	*quédese con el cambio*
keep this	*mantenga esto*
leave early	*salga temprano*
let me help you	*permítame ayudarle*
let's go take a break	*vamos a descansar*
let's see	*vamos a ver*
like this	*asi*
little by little	*poco a poco*

many things	*muchas cosas*
may be	*a lo mejor, ¡quizás!*
me neither	*yo tampoco*
merry christmas	*feliz navíidad*
more and more	*mas y mas*
more or less	*mas o menos*
my name is	*me llamo*
never!	*¡nunca!*
next year	*el año proximo*
not at all	*de ningún modo*
not so fast	*no tan rápido*
nothing	*nada*
of course (clearly)	*claro*
oh no!	*¡quiá!*
on an empty stomach	*con estómago vacío*
on call	*en guardia*
on one side	*por un lado*
on the other hand	*por otro iado*
once in a while	*de vez en cuando*
one a day (q.d.)	*una vez por día*
one moment (no more)	*¡un momento, no más!*
one more	*otromas*
outside	*afuera*
p.c.; after meals	*después de las comidas*
p.m. "at night"	*de la noche*
p.m. "in the afternoon"	*de la tarde*
p.o.; by mouth	*por la boca*
p.r.; by rectum	*en el recto*
pardon me, what did you say?	*¿mande?*
pardon; pardon me	*perdón; perdóneme usted*
pay now	*pague ahora*
phone me	*llámeme por teléfono*
please (beginning of a sentence)	*favor de…, …por favor*
please give me	*por favor, déme usted*
pleased to meet you ("enchanted")	*encantado,-a*
q.a.m.; when you get up in the morning	*cuando se levante por la mañana*
q.d; one a day	*una vez por día*
q.hs; before going to bed	*antes de acostarse*
q.i.d; four times a day	*cuatro veces al día*
q.o.d; every other day	*cada otra día*
relax	*relájese*
return in a week (in a month, etc.)	*vuelva en una semana (en un mes, etc.)*

right away (soon)	*¡pronto!*
rub this	*frotar esto*
see you later	*hasta la vista, hasta luego*
see you tomorrow	*nos vemos manana, hasta mañana*
show me	*muéstreme*
since when?	*¿de cuándo acá?*
sir, madam, miss	*señor, señora, señorita*
sit down, please	*siéntese, por favor*
smoking prohibited	*prohibido fumar*
so many things	*tantas cosas*
so much the better	*tanto mejor*
so much to see	*tanto que ver*
soak this	*remojar esto*
sold	*vendido*
some days in the hospital!	*¡unos días en el hospital!*
sometimes	*a veces*
speak slowly	*hable despacio*
stop	*¡pare!*
stop smoking	*deje de fumar*
stop!	*¡alto!*
suddenly	*de repente*
suffer from	*padece (padecido) de, sufre (sufrido) de*
swallow (pass saliva)	*pasa saliva*
swallow it	*tráguela*
t.i.d.; three times a day	*tres veces al día*
take (__) pills/tablets	*tome (__) pildoras/pastillas*
take a chill pill	*tome un resfrío pildora*
take care of yourself	*cuídese*
take this (ingest this)	*tome esto*
take this medicine	*tome esta medicina*
take this with food	*tome esto con comida*
tell me	*dígame*
thank you	*gracias*
thank you very much	*muchas gracias*
thanks "don't mention it"	*no hay de qué*
thanks "of nothing"	*de nada*
thanks for everything	*gracias por todo*
that happened	*eso pasa*
that's enough	*es suficiente*
that's interesting	*es interesante*
that's right	*es correno*
there he is	*alli esta él*
there is no cancer	*no hay cáncer*

there was, there were	habíal
think twice	plénselo bien
this one	éste
three times a day (t.i.d.)	tres veces al día
to the left	a la izquierda
to the right	a la derecha
to where?	¿a dónde?
to your health!	¡salud!
to your home!	¡a la casa!
turn left	doble a ia izquierda
turn right	doble a la derecha
unless	como no
until later/until I see you	hasta luego/hasta la vista
until the next appointment	hasta la próxima cita
until the next visit	hasta la próxima cita
usually	usualmente
very glad to have served you	muy contento en haberle servido
very good/well	muy bien
very well	muy bien
wait here	espere aquí
we all do the best we can	todo nosotros hace mos le mejor que podemos
we'll see	veremos
welcome	¡bienvenido!
well	bueno
what a pity	qué lástima
what color is your car?	¿de qué color es su coche?
what date?	¿qué fecha?
what day is it?	qué días es?
what do you think?	¿que piensa usted?
what does he say?	¿qué dice?
what else?	¿qué más?
what if?	¿y si?
what is he talking about?	¿de qué esta habiando?
what is your problem?	¿cuál es su problema?
what terrible weather	que mal tiempo
what time is it?	¿qué hora es?
what you're saying is irrelavent	lo que dice es impertinente
what's going on?	¿que pasa?
what's happening to you?	¿qué le pasa a usted?
what's the date today?	¿qué fecha es hoy?
what's the matter?	¿qué le pasa?
what?	¿qué?

when necessary	*cuando necesario*
when you get up in the morning (q.a.m.)	*cuando se levante por la mañana*
when?	*¿cuándo?*
where (whither)?	*¿a dónde?*
where are you going	*a dónde va usted*
where are you going?	*¿dónde va usted?*
where did this happen - the address	*dónde sucedió esto - la dirección*
where is my suitcase!?!	*¿dónde está mi maleta?*
where?	*¿dónde?*
which?	*¿cuál?*
who did it	*quién lo hizo*
who else?	*¿quién más?*
who is it?	*¿quién es?*
who is talking	*quién habla*
who?	*¿quién?*
why not?	*¿cómo no?, ¿por qué no?*
why?	*¿por qué?*
will you give me permission	*me da permiso*
with meals	*con las comidas*
with patience, one can gain heaven	*con paciencia se gana el cielo*
you are cured	*usted está curado*
you are going to live	*usted va a vivir*
you can go	*puede marcharse*
you have to come with me	*usted tiene que venir conmigo*
you have too	*usted hace*
you have too finish all of the medicine	*usted tiene que terminar toda la medicina*
you know him	*usted loconoce*
you look tired	*usted se ve cansado*
you mean	*usted quiere decir*
you musn't be afraid!	*¡no hay que llorar!*
you speak too fast	*usted habla demasiado*
you tell me and we'll both know	*usted digame y los dos llegaremos a saber*
you're crazy	*¡esta loco!*
you're early	*usted está adelantado*
you're here	*usted aqui*
you're kidding!	*esta bromeando*
you're lying	*está mintiendo*
you're too noisy	*demasiado ruido*
you're welcome	*de nada; no hay de qué*

COMMON POLICE VOCABULARY

answer my question	*conteste me pregunta*
answer yes or no	*conteste sí o no*
can you identify them	*puede identificarlos*
come here	*venga aquí, por favor*
come out with your hands up	*salga con las manos para arriba*
did you hear an explosion	*oyó una explosión*
did you start the fire	*empezó usted el incendio*
do you have a witness	*tiene testigos*
do you have any problems	*tiene usted algún problema*
do you have any weapons	*tiene algunas armas*
do you know who started the fire	*sabe quién empezó el incendio*
do you need a doctor	*necesita un médico/doctor*
do you speak english	*habla usted inglés*
don't get in the way	*quítese de en medio*
don't move	*no se mueva*
don't shoot	*no dispare*
dont' do that	*no haga eso*
drop that weapon	*suelte ese arma*
everybody out	*todos afuera*
everybody outside	*todos afuera*
fire	*fuego*
get going	*andele*
get out	*sálgase*
give me that	*déme eso*
give me the weapon	*déme el arma*
go home	*váyase a su casa*
go over there	*váyase para allá*
go that way	*vaya para allá*
help me	*ayúdeme*
help!	*socorro! ayuda!*
how many	*cuántos*
how old are you	*cuántos años tiene usted*
I know my rights	*yo sé mis derechos*
I'll be back	*yo regresaré*
Is everyone out	*salieron todos*
jump!	*Brinque!*
move back	*muévese para atrás*
slowly	*despacio*
stand back	*párese atrás*
stay here	*quédese aquí*
stay in the car	*quédese en el carro*

stay out	*quédese afuera*
we suspect arson	*sospechamos incendio premeditado*
what is her name	*cómo se llama ella*
what is his name	*cómo se llama él*
what is the victims name	*cuál es el nombre de la víctima*
where do you believe the fire started	*dónde cree que empezó el fuego*
who owns this house	*quién es dueño de esta casa*
you have the right to say nothing	*usted tiene el derecho de no decir nada*
you have the right to remain silent	*usted tiene el derech de permanecer callado*
anything you say can be used against you in a court of law	*calquier cosa que diga se puede usar contra usted en una corte de ley*
you have the right to consult with an attorney	*usted tiene el derecho de consultar con un abogado*
you have the right to have him present during your interrogation	*usted tiene el derecho tenerlo presente durante su interrogatirio*
if you want an attorney and you cannot afford one	*si usted quiere un abogado y no puede conseguirlo*
they can name one who can represent you before the interrogation	*se le puede nombrar uno para que le represente a usted antes del interrogatorio*
Do you understand each of these rights which I have explained to you	*Entiende usted cada uno de los derechos que you le he explicado*
Having these rights in mind	*Teniendo estos derechos en mente*
do you wish to speak with me now	*desea usted hablar conmigo ahora*
alcoholic	*alcohólico*
alien	*extranjero*
ambulance	*ambulancia*
armed	*armado*
assassin	*asesino*
attorney	*abogado*
bail	*fianza*
bandit	*bandito*
beggar	*limosnero*
black eye	*ojo amoratado*
black; race	*rasa negro*
border patrol	*patrulla de la frontera, patrulla fronteriza*
bully	*valentón, matón*
bum	*holgazán*

burglarize	*escalar para robar*
bystander	*espectador*
car; automobile	*coche, carro*
car; in a car	*en coche, en carro*
citizen	*ciudadno*
citizen; respectable	*ciudadno respetable*
coffin	*caja, ataúd*
color	*color*
constable	*guardia, policía*
corpse	*cadáver*
coward	*cobarde*
crazy	*loco*
criminal	*criminal*
cripple	*cojo, manco*
danger	*peligro*
death	*muerte*
deceased	*difunto*
delinquent	*delincuente, culpable*
derelict	*destruido*
detective	*detective*
divorce	*divorcio*
doctor	*doctor, médico*
drinker	*tomador*
driver's license	*licencia de manejar*
drug addict	*drogadicto*
drunk	*borracho*
employed	*empleado*
enemy	*enemigo*
escapee	*evadido, escapado*
felon	*felón*
fingerprinted (have prints taken)	*han tomando las huellas digitales*
first aid	*primeros auxilos*
gambler	*jugador*
gangster	*pistolero, gángster*
hijacked	*robado*
hitch-hiker	*autostopista*
hurt	*herido*
identification card	*tarjeta de identificación*
injured	*lastimado*
insane	*insano, loco*
jail	*cárcel*
jail break	*escaparse de cárcel*
jailer	*carcelero*

janitor	*mozo, portero*
judge	*juez*
justice of the peace	*juez de la paz*
lawyer	*licenciado*
liar	*mentiroso, embustero*
license	*licencia*
lost	*perdido*
malingerer, loiterer	*zanguango*
masked	*con máscara, enmascarado*
mayor	*alcalde*
minister	*ministro*
mole; on the face	*lunar*
murderer	*asesino, matador*
mystery	*misterio*
not armed	*no armado*
parents	*los padres*
passport	*pasaporte*
past record; has a bad record	*malos antecedentes, tiene mal record*
patrol wagon (truck)	*camión de policía*
pawn broker	*prestamista*
pimp	*palo blanco, alcahuete*
police	*polcía*
police brutality	*brutalidad por parte de la policía*
police chief	*jefe de policía*
probation	*probación*
probation officer	*oficial de probación*
prostitute	*protituta, puta, prostituta de calle, cantonera, callejera, golfa, carrerista*
prowler	*rondador, ladrón*
public defender	*defensor público*
public health official	*oficial de salubridad pública*
ring	*anillo*
rob (verb)	*robar*
run (verb)	*correr*
runaway	*fugitivo*
scar	*cicatriz*
sex	*sexo*
sex; to have sex	*tener relaciónes sexuales*
sheriff	*oficial de justicia*
shop-lifter	*ratero de tienda*
short	*bajo*
shot; having been shot	*tiro, disparo, balazo*
sign here	*firme aquí*

smelly	*apestoso, maloliente*
smuggler	*contrabandista*
stabbed	*puñolado*
steal (verb)	*robar*
streetwalker	*protituta, puta, prostituta de calle, cantonera, callejera, golfa, carrerista*
stupid	*estúpido*
suspect	*sospechoso*
tall	*alto*
tatoo	*tatuaje*
teenager (or 13 to 19 years of age)	*joven (de 13 a 19 años de edad)*
temper; bad	*mal genio*
tenant	*inquilino*
thief	*ladrón*
traffic officer	*oficial de tráfico*
truck	*camión*
unemployed	*sin empleo*
vagabond	*vagabundo*
visa	*visa*
wallet	*cartera, billetera*
warrant officer	*suboficial*
where-abouts	*dónde se halla*
where-abouts	*dónde se halla no se sabe*
white; race	*raza blanco*
with friends	*con amigos*
witnesses	*testigos*
wounded	*herido*
wretch	*canalla*
yellow; race	*raza oriental*
young	*joven*

LISTS - VOCABULARY

- CHIEF COMPLAINTS/SYMPTOMS
- ANATOMY/BODY PARTS
- VERBS & CONJUGATION
- VERB "TO BE" ET AL
- RELATIVES
- TIME/DATES/SEASONS
- FOODS
- OCCUPATIONS
- NUMBERS
- QUANTITY & AMOUNT
- COLORS
- INTERROGATIVES

SYMPTOMS/CHIEF COMPLAINTS

Doctor, I have...	*Doctor, yo tengo...*
Nurse, I have...	*Enfermera, yo tengo...*
Do you have or have you had at any time...	*Tiene o ha tenido alguna vez...*
Suffer from...	*Padece (Padecido) de...*
Suffer from...	*Sufre (Sufrido) de...*
Do you feel...	*Se Siente...*
Have you noticed...	*Ha notado...*
Do you have...	*Tiene...*
Have you had...	*Ha Tenido...*

Abscess	*Absceso*
Accident	*Accidente*
Accident-Bicycle	*Accidente De Bicicleta*
Accident-Car/Bus	*Accidente De Auto/Autobús*
Accident-Motocycle	*Accidente De Motocicleta*
Ache	*Achaque*
Ache-Back	*Dolor De Espalda*
Ache-Belly	*Dolor De Barriga*
Ache-Head	*Dolor De Cabeza*
Ache-Heart	*Angustia*
Ache-Stomach	*Dolor De Estómago/Cólicos*
Ache-Tooth	*Dolor De Muela/Dientes*
Addiction	*Adicción*
Allergies	*Alergia*
Amnesia "Loss of Memory"	*Pérdida De Memoria*
Anemia	*Anemia*
Anesthesia	*Anestesia*
Angina	*Angina*
Anxiety	*Ansiedad*
Appendicitis	*Apendicitis*
Appetite	*Apetito*
Arrhymia	*Arritmia*
Arthritis	*Artritis*
Asthma	*Asma*
Atherosclerosis	*Aterornatosis*
Backache	*Dolor De Espalda*
Belching	*Eructo/Regüeldo*
Belly Ache	*Dolor De Barriga*
Bite-Bee (Sting)	*Picadura De Abejas*
Bite-Cat	*Mordedura De Gato*
Bite-Dog	*Mordedura De Perro*
Bite-Flea	*Mordedura De Pulga*
Bite-Human	*Mordedura De Persona*
Bite-Mosquito	*Mordedura De Mollote*
Bite-Mosquito	*Mordedura De Mosquito*
Bite-Scorpion (sting)	*Picadura De Elalacran*
Bite-Snake	*Mordedura De Culebra*
Bite-Spider (Sting)	*Picadura De Araña*

Blackout	*Vísion Negra*
Bleeding	*Sangrado*
Bleeding Disorder	*Enfermedades hemorrágicas*
Bleeding Tendency	*Tendencia A Sangrar*
Blindness	*Ceguera*
Blisters ("Ampules")	*Ampolla*
Boil	*Divieso*
Bronchitis	*Bronquitis*
Bruise	*Moretón/Contusión*
Bullet Wound	*Balazo*
Bump/Lump	*Bulto/Protuberancia*
Burn	*Quemadura*
Bursitis	*Bursitis*
Cancer	*Cáncer*
Chest Pain	*Dolor En El Pecho*
Chickenpox	*Vericela*
Chills	*Escalofríos*
Choke	*Estrangulación*
Cirrhosis	*Cirrosis*
Cold Sore "Mouth Ulcers"	*Ulceras De La Boca*
Cold/Flu	*Resfriado/Gripe*
Confused	*Confundido*
Confusion	*Confusión*
Congestion	*Congestión*
Constipation	*Estreñimiento*
Convulsions	*Convulsións*
Cough	*Tos*
Cramps	*Calambres*
Crazy	*Loco*
Cut	*Cortada/Cortadura*
Cyanosis "Blue Skin"	*Piel Azulada*
Cyst	*Quiste*
Dandruff	*Caspa*
Deafness	*Sordera*
Dermatitis	*Dermatitis*
Diabetes	*Diabetes*
Diarrhea	*Diarrea*
Diptheria	*Difteria*
Discharge	*Secreciones/Desechos*
Discharge-Ear	*Desechos De Los Oídos*
Discharge-Penile	*Desechos De El Pene*
Discharge-Vaginal	*Flujó Vaginales*
Discharge-Vaginal	*Secreción Vaginal (Anormal)*
Discomfort	*Molestia*
Dizziness	*Mareo/Vértigo*
Drowsy	*Soñoliento/Modorro*
Drugs	*Drugas*
Drunk	*Borracho/Bolo*
Earwax (Cerumen)	*Cera, Cerilla*
Eczema	*Eczema*
Edema "Swelling Of Legs"	*Hinchazón De Las Piernas*
Embolism	*Embolismo*
Emotional	*Emocional*
Emphysema	*Enfisema*

Epilepsy	*Epilepsia*
Fainting Spell	*Desmayo*
Fart (Slang)	*Pedo*
Fear	*Miedo*
Fevers	*Fiebre/Calentura*
Fistula	*Fístula*
Flank Pian	*Dolor De Flanco/Lado*
Flu	*Gripe/Influenza*
Flushing (Blushing)	*Bochornos*
Fractures	*Fracturas*
Fungi	*Hongos*
Gall Bladder (Attack)	*Ataque De La Vesícular Biliar*
Gall Stones	*Cálculo Biliar or*
Gall Stones	*Piedras De La Hiel*
Gas	*Gas*
Gash	*Cuchillada*
Gastritis	*Gastritis*
German Measles	*Rubéola*
Glaucoma	*Glaucoma*
Goiter	*Bocio/Papera*
Gonorrhea	*Gonorrea*
Gout	*Gota*
Gunshot Wound	*Escopetazo*
Hair Loss	*Pérdida Del Pelo*
Hallucinations	*Alucinaciónes*
Handicap	*Impedimento*
Hay Fever	*Fiebre De Heno*
Headache	*Dolor De Cabeza*
Heart Ache	*Angustia*
Heart Attack	*Ataque Al Corazón*
Heart Broken	*Muerto De Pena*
Heart Burn	*Acedía*
Heart Disease	*Enfermedad Del Corazón*
Heart Failure	*Falla Cardiaca*
Heart Failure	*Falla Del Corazón*
Heart Murmur	*Soplo Del Corazón*
Hematchezia (Stool With Blood)	*Desposiones Con Sangre*
Hemetemesis (Vomit With Blood)	*Vómito Con Sangre*
Hemophilia	*Hemofilia*
Hemoptesis (Cough up blood)	*Tose Sangre*
Hemorrhage	*Hemorragia*
Hemorrhoids	*Almorranas*
Hepatitis	*Hepatitis*
Hernia	*Hernia*
Herpes	*Herpes*
Hiccups	*Hipo*
High Blood Pressure	*Alta Presión*
High Blood Sugar	*Alta Azúcar En La Sangre*
Hit/Punch	*Golpe/Pegar*
Hives (Urticaria)	*Urticaria/Ronchas*
Hoarseness	*Ronquera*
Hungry	*Hambre*
Hurt	*Duele*
Hypochondriac	*Hipocondriáco*

Illness	*Enfermedad*
Immunization	*Immunización*
Impotence	*Impotencia*
Indigestion	*Indigestion*
Infection	*Infección*
Infectious Mononucleosis	*Mononucleosis Infecciosa*
Ingrown Nail	*Uñero*
Injury	*Daño/Herida*
Insanity	*Locura*
Insomnia	*Insomnio*
Itch	*Picazón/Comezón*
Jaundice ("Yellow Skin")	*Piel Amarilla/Ictericia*
Jones	*Adicción De Basquetbol*
Kidney "Rock"	*Piedra En El Riñón*
Kidney Disease	*Enfermedad de los riñones*
Kidney Stone	*Cálculo En El Riñón*
Kidney Stone "Stone Sickness"	*Mal De Piedra*
Laceration	*Laceración*
Lacrimation/Tearing	*Lágrimación/Lágrimas*
Lactation	*Lactación*
Lame	*Cojo*
Laryngitis	*Laringitis*
Leukemia	*Leucemia*
Lice	*Piojos*
Liver Disease	*Enfermedad del hígado*
Loss Of Conciousness	*Perdida Del Conocimiento*
Lung Disease	*Enfermedades pulmones*
Malaria	*Malaria*
Malignancy	*Malignidad*
Malnutrition	*Mala Nutrición*
Manic-Depressive	*Maniacodepresivo*
Measles	*Sarampión*
Meningitis	*Meningitis*
Menopause	*Menopausia*
Mental Illness	*Enfermedades mentales*
Migraine	*Migraña/Jaqueca*
Mite	*Ácaro*
Mole	*Lunar*
Multiple Sclerosis	*Esclerosis Múltiple*
Mumps	*Paperas*
Muscular Dystrophy	*Distrofia Muscular*
Mute	*Mudo*
Myalgia	*Dolor De Músculo*
Myocardial Infart	*Infarto Miocardíaco*
Myopia	*Miopia*
Nasal Congestion	*Congestión Nasal*
Nausea	*Náusea*
Nephritis	*Nefritis*
Nervousness	*Nervioso*
Neuralgia	*Neuralgia*
Night Sweats	*Sudores En La Noche*
Nocturia "...During The Night"	*Orinas Durante La Noche*
Numb	*Dormido*

Numbness	*Adormecimiento*
Obese	*Obeso*
Obstruction	*Obstrucción*
Osteomyelitis	*Osteromielitis*
Overdose	*Sobredosis*
Pain	*Dolor*
Pain-Boring	*Dolor Penetrante*
Pain-Burning	*Dolor Que Quema*
Pain-Continuous	*Dolor Continuo*
Pain-Cramping	*Dolor Calambre*
Pain-Deep	*Dolor Hondo*
Pain-Dull	*Dolor Sordo*
Pain-Gripping	*Dolor Resgante*
Pain-Heavy	*Dolor Pesado*
Pain-Intense	*Dolor Intensivo*
Pain-Intermittent	*Dolor Intermitente*
Pain-Labor	*Dolor Del Parto*
Pain-Light/Moderate	*Dolor Ligero/Moderado*
Pain-Pressure	*Dolor Con Presión*
Pain-Referred	*Dolor Referido*
Pain-Ripping	*Dolor Rasgante*
Pain-Severe	*Dolor Severo/Fuertes*
Pain-Sharp	*Dolor Agudo*
Pain-Shooting	*Dolor Punzante*
Pain-Tearing	*Dolor Desgarrante*
Pain-That Moves	*Dolor Que Se Mueve*
Pain-Throbbing	*Dolor Pulsante*
Pain-Tightness	*Dolor Tirantez*
Palpitation	*Palpitación*
Palsy	*Parálisis*
Pancreatitis	*Pancreatitis*
Paralysis	*Parálisis*
Paralysis-Cerebral	*Parálisis Cerebral*
Paralysis-Facial	*Parálisis Facial*
Parasthesias	*Sensaciones Inusuales En Su Piel*
Parkinson's Disease	*Enfermedad De Parkinson*
Peptic Ulcer	*Úlcera Peptica*
Pertussis	*Tos Convulsiva*
Phlegm	*Flema*
Pimple	*Grano/Barro*
Pleurisy	*Pleuresia*
Pneumonia	*Pulmonía*
Poison	*Ponzoña/Veneno*
Polio	*Poliomielitis*
Polydypsia "Thirsty All The Time"	*Sed/Sediento Todo El Tiempo*
Polyp	*Pólipo*
Polyuria "Urinate with frequency"	*Orinas con frecuencia*
Pregnant	*Encinta/Embarazada*
Problem	*Problema/Trastorno*
Psoriasis	*Psoríasis*

Psychosis	Psicosis
Pus	Pus
Pyorhhea	Piorrea
Rabies	Rabia
Rash	Salpullido/Erupción
Redeye	Ojo Rojo
Relapse	Recaída
Retardation	Retardación
Rheumatic Fever	Fiebre Reumática
Ringing In Ears	Zumbido
Ringworm (Tinea)	Tiña
Roseola	Roséola
Rubella	Rubéola
Runny Nose	Catarra/Moquean
Sea Sick	Mareo
Scab	Costra
Scabies	Sarna
Scar	Cicatriz
Scarlet Fever	Escarlatina
Scratch	Raspón/Rasguño
Seizures	Convulsiones/Ataques
Senility	Senil
Sensation	Sensación
Shock	Choque
Sick	Enfermo/Malo
Sigh	Suspiro
Skin-Cracked	Grieta
Skin-Discolored	Paños
Skin-Dry	Piel Seca
Skin-Irritaion	Irritación De La Piel
Skin-Oily	Piel Grasosa
Smallpox	Viruela
Sneeze	Estornudo
Sore	Llaga
Sore Throat	Dolor De Garganta
Spasm	Espasmo
Spotting	Manchanas/Coágulos
Sprain	Torcedura
Stab Wound	Puñalada
Stiff	Tieso
Stitches/Sutures	Puntadas/Puntos
Stomach Ache	Cólicos
Stomach Ache	Dolor De Estómago
Strabismus	Estabismo, Ojos Cruz
"No Control In One Eye"	Sin Control En Un Ojo
Strain	Torcedura
Stress/Tension	Tensión
Stroke	Apoplejía/Derrame Cerebral
Sty	Orzuelo
Suffocation	Sofocación

Suicide	*Suicidio*
Sunburn	*Quemadura De Sol*
Surgery	*Cirugía*
Sweating	*Sudor*
Swelling	*Hinchazón*
Symptom	*Síntoma*
Syphyilis	*Sífilis*
Tachycardia	*Taquicardia*
Tetanus	*Tétanos*
Thirst	*Sed*
Thyroid Problems	*Problemas de la tiroides*
Tingling	*Hormigueo*
Tonsillitis	*Tonsilitis*
Toothache	*Dolor De Muela/Dientes*
Trauma	*Trauma*
Tremble	*Tremblor*
Trembling	*Temblor*
Tuberculosis (TB)	*Tuberculosis*
Tumor	*Tumor*
Twitch/Tic	*Crispatura/Tremblor*
Typhoid Fever	*Fiebre Tifoidea*
Typhus	*Tifus*
Ulcer	*Úlcera*
Unconciousness	*Insensibilidad/Inconsiente*
Urine-Dark	*Orin Oscuro*
Urine-Pain	*Dolor Al Orinar*
Varicose Veins	*Venas Varicosas*
Venereal Disease	*Enfermedad Venérea*
Victim	*Víctim*
Virus	*Virus*
Vision-Blurred	*Vista Nublada*
Vision-Double	*Vista Doble*
Vision/View	*Visión/Vista*
Vomiting	*Vómito*
Wart	*Verruga*
Weakness	*Debilidad/Débil*
Weight Change	*Cambiado De Peso*
Welt/Wheal	*Roncha*
Wheeze	*Silbar/Jadear*
Whiplash "Neck Injury"	*Lastimado Del Cuello*
Worms	*Lombrices*
Worried	*Preocupado*
Wound	*Herida*
Yellow Fever	*Fiebre Amarilla*

Cultural Note: "Derecha" is the Spanish word for "Right" (as opposed to "Left"). However a similar word, "Derecho," is the word for "Straight Ahead." Depending upon context, "Derecho" can also mean "Right" as in "Bill of Rights" or "Law" as in "Criminal Law" ("Derecho Penal"). As you can imagine, this can become very difficult to determine which meaning is inferred if your knowledge of Spanish is limited.

ANATOMY/BODY PARTS/BODY REGIONS

Areas:

Head	Cabeza
Face	Cara/Rostro
Back	Espalda
Belly	Panza/Barriga
Abdomen	Vientre
Chest	Pecho
Breasts	Senos

HEENT:

Beard	Barba
Cheek	Cachete
Chin	Barbilla
Ears	Oídos/Orejas
Eustacion Tube	Tubo De Eustaquin
Eyebrow	Ceja
Eyelash	Pestaña
Eyelid	Párpado
Eyes	Ojos
Face	Rostro/Cara
Forehead	Frente
Freckles	Pecas
Jaw	Mejilla
Lips	Labios
Mouth	Boca
Mustache	Bigote
Neck	Cuello
Nose	Nariz
Nostril	Fosa Nasal
Pupil	Pupila
Sinus	Seno
Tear	Lágrima
Teeth	Dientes
Temple	Sien
Throat	Garganta
Tongue	Lengua
Wrinkles	Arrugas
Zygoma	Cigomatica
Adam's Apple	La Nuez de Adam (Adan)

Specific Anatomy

Heart	Corazón
Lungs	Pulmones
Liver	Hígado
Kidneys	Riñones
Spleen	Bazo
Skin	Piel

Anus	*Ano*
Appendix	*Apéndice*
Bladder	*Vejiga*
Bronchi	*Bronquios*
Brain	*Cerebro*
Buttocks	*Cadera/Nalgas*
GallBladder	*Vesícula Biliar*
Hair	*Pelo/Cabello*
Intestines	*Intestino*
Nerves	*Nervios*
Pancreas	*Páncreas*
Penis	*Pene*
Rectum	*Recto*
Stomach	*Estómago*
Scapula	*Escápula*
Vagina	*Vagina*
Womb	*Matriz*

Extremities/Orthopedics

Bones	*Huesos*
Arms	*Brazos*
Shoulder	*Hombro*
Clavicle	*Clavícula/"Hueso del cuello"*
Joints	*Articulación*
Muscles	*Músculos*
Hips/Buttocks	*Cadera*
Elbow/Forearm	*Codo/Antebrazo*
Hands	*Manos*
Fingers	*Dedos*
Fingernail	*Uñas*
Thumb	*Pulgar/Dedo Gordo*
Wrists	*Muñecas*
Palm	*Palms*
Legs	*Piernas*
Knee	*Rodillas*
Knee Bone/Patella	*Hueso De La Rodilla/Rótula*
Calves	*Pantorrillas*
Shin	*Espinilla*
Feet	*Pies*
Ankle	*Tobillos*
Toes	*Dedos Del Pie*
Heel/Sole	*Talón/Planta Del Pie*
Fracture	*Quebradura/Fractura*
	/Rotura de hueso
Bowlegged	*Corvo*
Corns	*Callos*
Flat Foot	*Pie Plano*
Sprain	*Torcedura/"Falsiado"*
Dislocate	*Dislocar/Descoyuntar*

> **Cultural Note:** "Nalgas," although a correct word for "hips," it is considered vulgar. In English, it roughly translates into "ass." The preferred word for hips/buttocks is "cadera."

VERBS - REGULAR VERBS

Each complete sentence in Spanish must contain a subject and a verb.

Irregular verbs are verbs which need to be conjugated specifically for each subject, therefore they are called, "Irregular" (and are not addressed here).

Regular verbs are verbs which can be conjugated by a predetermined set of rules, therefore they are called "Regular." They contain a stem (or root) whose ending can be modified to suit the subject of the sentence.

There are three basic forms of regular verbs in Spanish. Each ends with a unique two-letter combination:

"-ar"	e.g.	Hablar (to speak)
"-er"	e.g.	Caer (to fall)
"-ir"	e.g.	Salir (to come out)

CONJUGATE (-AR), (-ER), (-IR) REGULAR VERBS

VERB ENDINGS*		-AR	-ER	-IR
I	(Yo)	-o	-o	-o
You	(Usted)	-as	-es	-es
You Pleural	(Usted)	-an	-en	-en
He/She	(El/Ella)	-a	-e	-e
We	(Nosotros)	-amos	-emos	-emos
They	(Ellos/Ellas)	-an	-en	-ir

* Change the ending of the verb according to the subject.

Take for example, the verb "Lavar" (to wash)

VERB ENDINGS		-AR
I	(Yo)	lav-o
You	(Usted)	lav-as
You Pleural	(Usted)	lav-an
He/She	(El/Ella)	lav-a
We	(Nosotros)	lav-amos
They	(Ellos/Ellas)	lav-an

TO BE - *THE VERB*

PRONOUN

I	**Yo**
He	Él
She	Élla
You (Singular)	Usted
You (Pleural)	Ustedes
They (Masculine)	Ellos
They (Feminine)	Ellas

TO BE

I am	Soy
He is	Él es
She is	Ella es
We are	Nosotros somos
You (Singular) are	Usted es
You (Pleural) are	Ustedes son
They (Masculine) are	Ellos son
They (Feminine) are	Ellas son

TO HAVE

I have	Yo **Tengo**
He has	El **Tiene**
She has	Ella Tiene
We have	Nosotros tenemos
You (Singular) have	Usted tiene
You (Pleural) have	Ustedes tienen
They (Masculine) have	Ellos tienen
They (Feminine) have	Ellas tienen

TO WANT

I want	Yo quiero
He wants	El quiere
She wants	Ella quiere
We want	Nosotros queremos
You (Singular) want	Usted quiere
You (Pleural) want	Ustedes quieren
They (Masculine) want	Ellos quieren
They (Feminine) want	Ellas quieren`

RELATIVES

Wife	*Esposa/Mujer*
Husband	*Esposo/Marido*
Mother	*Madre/Mamá*
Father	*Padre/Papá*
Sister/Brother	*Hermana/Hermano*
Daughter/ Son	*Hija/ Hijo*
Aunt/Uncle	*Tía/Tío*
Grandmother	*Abuela*
Grandfather	*Abuelo*
Granddaughter	*Nieta*
Grandson	*Nieto*
Cousin (F/M)	*Prima/Primo*
Woman/Man	*Mujer/Hombre*
Child-Girl/Boy	*Niña/Niño*
Mother-In-Law	*Suegra*
Father-In-Law	*Suegro*
Sister-In-Law	*Cuñada*
Brother-In-Law	*Cuñado*
Daughter-In-Law	*Nuera*
Son-In-Law	*Yerno*
Friend (F/M)	*Amiga/Amigo*
Family	*Familia*
Niece/Nephew	*Sobrina/Sobrino*
Parents	*Los Padres*
Stepmother	*Madrastra*
Stepfather	*Padrastro*
Stepdaughter	*Alnada/Hijastra*
Stepson	*Alnado/Hijastro*
Godmother	*Madrina*
Godfather	*Padrino*

La Madre + El Padre	*Los Padres*
La Hermana + El Hermano	*Los Hermanos*
Mister (Mr.)	*Senor (Sr.)*
Misses (Mrs.)	*Senora (Sra.)*
Miss (Miss)	*Senorita (Srta.)*

Cultural Note: "Mujer" (woman) can also be used to refer to a common law wife.

MONTHS/DAY/YEAR

Seconds	*Segundos*
Minutes	*Minutos*
Hours	*Horas*
Days	*Días*
Weeks	*Semanas*
Months	*Meses*
Years	*Años*

Before	*Antes (de)*
During	*Durante*
After	*Después (de)*
Until	*Hasta*
At (Time)	*A Las*
Always	*Siempre*
Never	*Nunca*
Right Now (Stat)	*Ahora Mismo*
Now	*Ahora*
Soon	*Pronto*
Earlier	*Más Temprano*
Later	*Más Tarde*
Past	*Pasado*
Last	*Ultimo*
Next	*Próximo*
Since	*Desde*
Date	*Fecha*

Yesterday	*Ayer*
Today	*Hoy*
Tomorrow	*Mañana*
Day Before Last	*Anteayer*
Day After Next	*Pasado Mañana*
Morning	*en la Mañana*
Noon	*Medio Dias*
Afternoon	*La Tarde*
Midnight	*Medianoche*
Tonight	*Esta Noche*
Night	*Noche*
Last Night	*Anoche*

Time	*Tiempo*
On Time	*A Tiempo*
Times (occasions)	*Vez*
Wait	*Espere*

Ago	"*Hace*" + reference of time. For example, "two days ago" would be "*hace dos días*"
How Long Ago	*Hace cuánto tiempo*

DAYS OF THE WEEK

Monday	*Lunes*
Tuesday	*Martes*
Wednesday	*Miércoles*
Thursday	*Jueves*
Friday	*Viernes*
Saturday	*Sábado*
Sunday	*Domingo*

MONTHS

January	*Enero*
February	*Febrero*
March	*Marzo*
April	*Abril*
May	*Mayo*
June	*Junio*
July	*Julio*
August	*Agosto*
September	*Septiembre*
October	*Octubre*
November	*Noviembre*
December	*Diciembre*

SEASONS

Spring	*Primavera*
Summer	*Verano/Estival*
Fall/Autumn	*Ontoño*
Winter	*Inverno*

PHRASES

AM "In the morning"	*De la mañana*
PM "At night"	*De la noche*
PM "In the afternoon"	*De la tarde*
Today is Monday	*Hoy es lunes*
Tomorrow is Monday	*Mañana es lunes*
What day is it?	*¿Qué días es?*
What day is it today?	*¿Qué día es hoy?*
What time is it?	*¿Qué hora es?*
Yesterday was Monday	*Ayer fue lunes*
What is the date?	*¿Cuál es la fecha?*
What month is this?	*¿En qué mes estamos?*
It's one o'clock	*Es la una*
It's two o'clock	*Son las dos*
It's two-thirty	*Son las dos y media*

Cultural Note: In Spanish, you do not say, "I'll see you in a week;" you say, "I'll see you in 8 days." Two weeks is 15 days. If you say, "I'll see you in 14 days," your patient may get confused and show up a day early.

FOODS

Food	*Alimento/Comida*
Diet	*Dieta*
Calories	*Calorías*
Vitamins	*Vitaminas*
Breakfast	*Desayuno*
Lunch	*Almuerzo*
Dinner	*Cena/Comida*
To Starve	*Hambrear*
Feed	*Alimentarse*
Nothing By Mouth (NPO)	*Nada para la boca*

MEATS	*CARNES*
Bacon	*Tocino*
Beef	*Carne De Vaca*
Chicken	*Pollo*
Duck	*Pato*
Ham	*Jamón*
Hamburger	*Hamburguesa*
Fish	*Pescado*
Fowl	*Ave*
Lamb	*Cordero*
Liver	*Hígado*
Meat	*Carne*
Pork	*Carne De Puerco*
Sausage	*Chorizo*
Steak	*Biftec*
Turkey	*Pavo*

METHOD	*MÉTODO*
Baked	*Al Hornoa*
Barbecue	*Barbacoa*
Boiled	*Hervido*
Broiled	*A La Parrilla*
Cook	*Cocer/Cocinar*
Fillet	*Filete*
Fried/Fry	*Frito/Freír*
Roasted	*Asado*
Sandwich	*Sandwich*

VEGETABLE	LEGUMBRES
Bean (South America)	Habichuela
Bean (Mexico)	Los Frijoles
Beet	Remolecha
Carrot	Zanahoria
Celery	Apio
Corn	Maíz
Cucumber	Pepino
Lettuce	Lechuga
Onion	Cebolla
Potato	Patata
Rice	Arroz
Salad	Ensalada
Spinach	Espinaca
Tomato	Tomate
Vegetable	Legumbre
Yam	Batata

FRUITS	FRUTAS
Apple	Manzana
Banana	Banana
Canteloupe	Cantalupo
Citrus Fruits	Agruras
Fruit	Fruta
Grape	Uva
Grapefruit	Toronja
Lemon	Limón
Melon	Melón
Nut	Nuez
Orange	Naranja
Peach	Melocotón
Pear	Pera
Prune	Ciruela Pasa
Strawberry	Fresa
Tomato	Tomate
Watermelon	Sandír

BREAD/GRAIN	PAN/GRANOS
Bread	Pan
Cake	Torta/Pastel
Cookie	Gelleta Dulce
Cracker	Galleta
Flour (Corn)/(Wheat)	Harina (De Maíz)/(De Trigo)
Grain	Granos
Pie	Pastel
Roll	Panecillo
Tortilla	Tortilla
Wheat	Trigo

DAIRY	LECHERIA
Butter	Mantequilla
Cheese	Queso
Cream	Crema
Egg	Huevo
Ice Cream	Helado
Lard	Manteca
Milk (of Cows)	Leche (De Vaca)
Raw Milk	Leche Fresca
Skim Milk	Leche Descremada
Powder Milk	Leche En Polvo
Yogurt	Yogurt

SEASONING/OILS/ETC	ADEREZO/ACEITE/ETC
Catsup	Salsa de tomate
Chocolate	Chocolate
Dessert	Postre
Jam	Mermelada
Jelly	Jelea
Mayonnaise	Mayonesa
Mustard	Mostaza
Oil	Aceite
Pepper	Pimienta
Salt	Sal
Salad Dressing	Salsa/Aliño
Sugar	Azúcar
Sweets/Candy	Dulces/Bombóm
Vanilla	Vainilla

LIQUIDS	LIQUIDOS
Beer	Cerveza
Coffee	Café
Juice	Jugo
Liquids	Líquidos
Liquour	Licor
Soda	Soda
Soup	Sopa, caldo
Tea	Té
Water	Agua
Whiskey	Whiskey "We-Ski"
Wine	Vino "Vee-No"

I'm hungry...	Tengo hambre...	I would like...	Me gustaría...
I'm thirsty...	Tengo sed...	I want...	Quisiera...
I need...	Necisito...	Can I Have...	¿Puedo Tener...?

OCCUPATIONS, A RANDOM ASSORTMENT

Doctor (M.D.)	*Médico*
Doctor (PhD or M.D.)	*Doctor*
Nurse	*Enfermera*
Surgeon	*Cirujano*
Resident	*Residente*
Intern	*Interno*
Paramedic	*Paramédico*
Pharmacist	*Farmacéutico*
Medical Student	*Estudiante de medicina*
Dentist	*Dentista*
Obstetrician	*Partero*
Midwife/Wet nurse	*Partera/Nodriza*
Banker	*Banquero*
Barber	*Peluquero, barbero*
Businessman	*Comerciante*
Butcher	*Carnicero*
Carpenter	*Carpintero*
Clergy	*Pastor/Clérigo*
Cook	*Cocinero*
Druggist	*Boticario, droguista*
Engineer	*Ingeniero*
Farmer	*Hacendado, agricultor*
Fireman	*Bombero*
Fisherman	*Pescador*
Gardener	*Jardinero*
Guide	*Guía*
Harvester	*Cosechero*
Housewife	*Ama de casa*
Lawyer	*Abogado, licenciado*
Machinist	*Maquinista*
Mechanic	*Mecánico*
Musician	*Músico*
Painter	*Pintor*
Picker (of crops)	*Piscador*
Planter	*Plantador, sembrador*
Plumber	*Plomero*
Policeman	*Policía*
Priest	*Cura, sacerdote, padre*
Rancher	*Ranchero*
Secretary	*Secrétario*
Sheriff	*Alguacil, policía*
Teacher	*Profesor, maestro, Instructor*
Waiter	*Mozo, mesero, camarero*
Working Man	*Trabajor/Obrer*
Working Woman	*Trabajora/Obrera*

NUMBERS

Card	Ord	Cardinals	Ordinals
0	0th	*Cero*	————
1	1st	*Uno (1)*	*Primero (1°)*
2	2nd	*Dos (2)*	*Segundo (2°)*
3	3rd	*Tres (3)*	*Tercero (3°)*
4	4th	*Cuatro*	*Cuarto(4°)*
5	5th	*Cinco*	*Quinto (5°)*
6	6th	*Seis*	*Sexto*
7	7th	*Siete*	*Séptimo*
8	8th	*Ocho*	*Octavo*
9	9th	*Nueve*	*Noveno*
10	10th	*Diez*	*Décimo*
11	11th	*Once*	*Undécimo*
12	12th	*Doce*	*Duodécimo*
13	13th	*Trece*	*Décimo Tercio*
14	14th	*Catorce*	*Décimo Cuarto*
15	15th	*Quince*	*Décimo Quinto*
16	16th	*Dieci-Séis*	*Décimo Sexto*
17	17th	*Dieci-Siete*	*Décimo Séptimo*
18	18th	*Dieci-Ocho*	*Décimo Octavo*
19	19th	*Dieci-Nueve*	*Décimo Nono*
20	20th	*Veinte*	*Vigésimo*
21	21st	*Viente y Uno*	*Vigésimo Primo*
22	22nd	*Viente y Dós*	*Vigésimo Segundo*
23	23rd	*Viente y Trés*	*Vigésimo Tercero*
24	24th	*Viente y Cuatro*	*Vigésimo Cuarto*
25	25th	*Viente y Cinco*	*Vigésimo Quinto*
30	30th	*Treinta*	*Trigésimo*
31	31st	*Treinta y Uno*	*Trigésimo Primo*
40	40th	*Cuarenta*	*Cuardragésimo*
50	50th	*Cincuenta*	*Quincuagésimo*
60	60th	*Sesenta*	*Sexagésimo*
70	70th	*Setenta*	*Septuagésimo*
80	80th	*Ochenta*	*Octogésimo*
90	90th	*Noventa*	*Nonagésimo*
100	100th	*Cien*	*Centésimo*
101	101st	*Ciento-Uno*	
100+		*Ciento+Etc...*	
200		*Doscientos*	*Ducentésimo*
300		*Trescientos*	*Trecentésimo*
400		*Cuatrocientos*	*Cuadragentésimo*
500		*Quinientos*	*Quingentésimo*
600		*Seiscientos*	*Sexcentésimo*
700		*Setecientos*	*Septegentésimo*
800		*Ochocientos*	*Octogentésimo*
900		*Novecientos*	*Nonagentésimo*

1000	*Mil*	*Milésimo*
1990	*Mil Novencientos Noventa*	
1991	*Mil Novencientos Noventa Y Uno*	
1992	*Mil Novencientos Noventa Y Dos*	
1993	*Mil Novencientos Noventa Y Tres*	
1994	*Mil Novencientos Noventa Y Cuatro*	

QUANTITY/COMPARISONS

All	*Todo*
None	*Nada/Ninguno*
Neither	*Ninguno*
Half	*Medio*
A Few (Some)	*Unas*
A Lot	*Mucho*
Very Much	*Muchísimo*
Little	*Un Poco*
Very Little	*Un Poquito*
More	*Más*
Less	*Menos*
Most	*La Major Parte*
Least	*Menor/Mínimo*
Enough/Sufficient	*Bastante*
Plenty	*Completamente*
Too Much	*Demasiado*
Better	*Mejor*
Worse	*Peor*

AMOUNTS

Teaspoon	*Cucharita*
Tablespoon	*Cuchara*
Cupful	*Taza*
Quart	*Cuarto*
Gallon	*Galón*
Pound	*Libra*
Ounce	*Onza*
Inch	*Pulgada*
Foot	*Pie*
Yard	*Yarda*
Mile	*Milla*
Meter	*Metro*
Kilometer	*Kilómetro*

COLORS   LOS COLORES

Black	*Negro*
Copper	*Cobre*
Beige	*Beige, Amarillento*
Cream	*Crema, Perla*
Maroon	*Marrón*
Olive	*Olivo*
Tan	*Café Claro*
Turquoise	*Turquesa*
Blue	*Azul*
Brown	*Moreno, Café, Pardo*
Gold	*Dorado*
Grey	*Gris*
Green	*Verde*
Orange	*Anaranjado, Naranja*
Pink	*Rosado, Rosa*
Purple	*Purpura*
Violet	*Morado, Violeta*
Red	*Rojo, Colorado*
Silver	*Plateado*
White	*Blanco*
Yellow	*Amarillo*

HAIR COLORS/MODIFIERS

Clear	*Claro*
Dark	*Oscuro*
Light	*Claro*
Natural	*Natural*
Transparent	*Transparente*
Blonde	*Rubio*
Brunette	*Moreno*
Grey Hair	*Canas*

What color is your...	*De qué color es su...*
What was the color of...	*De qué color era el/la...*
Do you remember the color?	*¿Recuerda usted el color?*

INTERROGATIVES

Who	*¿Quién?*
What	*¿Qué?*
When	*¿Cuándo?*
Where	*¿Dónde?*
Why	*¿Por Qué?*
Which	*¿Cuál?*
How	*¿Cómo?*

For what reason?	*¿Por dónde?*
From where?	*¿De dónde?*
How come/Since when?	*¿De cuándo acá?*
How do you say ____?	*¿Cómo se dice ____?*
How Far	*¿Hasta Dónde?*
How Long (time)	*¿Cuánto Tiempo?*
How Many	*¿Cuántos?*
How Much	*¿Cuánto?*
How much is...?	*¿A cómo es...?*
How Often	*¿Cuántas Veces?*
How often do you... ?	*¿Qué tan seguido...?*
How Old	*¿Cuántas Años?*
How's everything?	*¿Qué tal?*
Unless...	*Como no...*
What Date	*¿Qué Fecha?*
What Else	*¿Qué Más?*
What If...	*¿Y Si...?*
Whither (to where)?	*¿A dónde?*
Who Else	*¿Quién Más?*
Why not?	*¿Cómo no?*
Why not?	*¿Por qué no?*

Oh No!	*¡Quiá!*
Maybe!	*¡Quizás!*
Already!	*¡Ya!*

Spanish Note: Interogatives can often be confusing. "Cómo," according to the dictionary definition, can mean *how, why,* or *what*. I've only given the most common meaning of the classic interogatives in this section.

SIGNS/DIRECTIONS

Right	*Derecha*
Left	*Izquierda*
Straight	*Recto/Derecho*
Along here	*Por aji*
Around here	*Por aquí*
Can you tell me...?	*¿Me puede decir...?*
Go straight ahead	*Siga derecho*
Here	*Aquí*
Is it far?	*¿Está lejos?*
Turn left	*Doble a ia izquierda*
Turn right	*Doble a la derecha*
Where is...?	*¿Dónde esta...?*
Bathing Prohibited	*Prohibido bañarse*
Cashier	*Caja*
Caution	*Cuidado*
Closed	*Cerrado*
Cold	*Frío/"F"*
Danger	*Peligro*
Don't touch	*No tocar*
Down	*Abajo*
Elevator	*Ascensor*
Entrance	*Entrada*
Entry prohibited	*Prohibido el paso*
Exit	*Salida*
For Rent	*Se alquila*
For Sale	*Se vende*
Hot & Cold	*Caliente & Frío/"C" & "F"*
Ladies Room	*Damas/Señoras*
Mens Room	*Caballeros/Hombres*
Occupied	*Ocupado*
Open	*Abierto*
Parking prohibited	*Prohibido aparcar/estacionamiento*
Pull	*Tirar*
Push	*Empujar*
Reserved	*Reservado*
Restrooms	*Lavabos/Servicios*
Smoking prohibited	*Prohibido fumar*
Spitting prohibited	*Prohibido escupir*
Stop	*Alto*
Up	*Arriba*
Vacant	*Libre*
Walk (Crosswalk)	*Pase*
Walking on grass prohibited	*Prohibido pisar el césped*

THE DICTIONARY

- **MEDICAL SPANISH**
- **COMMON USAGE SPANISH**

- In order to facilitate your education, I've created a general use Spanish dictionary. When I completed the original version, it was over 2,500 words, mainly medical Spanish. I then turned my attention to include more commonly used words. The end result was a dictionary with over 6,500 entries.

- You will find that learning Spanish is more a course in expanding your English vocabulary than in learning an entire new language. Many Spanish words are derived from the same Latin roots which are common in English.

- When more than one Spanish word is given for a single English listing, no preference is given to the available choices. For example, menstrual period is given as "regla" and "menstruación." There is no preference. You may simple have to try both phrases and see which is more accepted by your patient population.

- As a common useage dictionary, you may find it useful when traveling to a Spanish speaking country.

- Regardless of the number of phrases available, you will run into circumstances which requires vocabulary beyond the scope of the phrases and vocabulary presented here.

A

a lot: *mucho*

a.c.; before meals: *antes de las comidas*

a.i.d.s.; acquired immune deficiency syndrome: *s.i.d.a., síndrome de immunidad deficiente adquirida*

a.m.: *ante maridiem*

a.s.a.p.: *cuanto antes, lo más pronto posible*

abandon (v.): *abandonar*

abbot: *abad*

abbreviation: *abreviatura*

abdicate (v.): *abdicar*

abdomen: *vientre, abdomen*

ability: *habilidad*

abnormal: *anormal*

abnormality: *anormalidad*

aboard: *a bordo*

abominable: *abominable, pésimo*

abortion: *aborto*

abortion; induced: *aborto provocado, aborto inducido, aborto voluntario*

abortion; spontaneous: *malparto, aborto involuntario, aborto accidental*

abortion; therapeutic: *aborto terapéutico*

abound (v.): *abundar*

about: *acerca de, alrededor, cosa de, de*

above: *arriba, sobre, encima de*

abrasion: *razpón, rozadura*

abrupt: *brusco, abrupto*

abscess: *absceso*

absence: *ausencia*

absent-minded: *distraído*

absent: *ausente*

absolve (v.): *absolver*

absorb (v.): *absorber*

absorption: *absorción*

abstain (v.): *abstener(se)*

abstinence: *abstinencía*

abstract (v.): *abstraer*

abstraction: *abstracción*

absurd: *absurdo*

absurdity: *ridiculez*

abundance: *abundancia*

abundant: *abundante*

abuse (v.): *abusar de, ajar*

abuse: *maltrato*

abuse; child: *maltrato de los niños*

abyss: *abismo*

academy: *academia*

accent (v.): *acentuar*

accent: *acento, dejo*

accept (v.): *aceptar*

acceptable: *aceptable*

access: *acceso*

accessible: *accesible*

accident: *accidente, atropello*

accident; bicycle: *accidente de bicicleta*

accident; bus: *accidente de autobús*

accident; car: *accidente de auto*

accident; motocycle: *accidente de motocicleta*

acclaim (v.): *aclamar*

acclimatize (v.): *aclimatar*

according to: *de aceuado con, según*

account: *cuenta, reseña*

accounting: *contaduría*

accumulate (v.): *acaudalar, acumular*

accurate: *exacto*

accuse (v.): *acusar, inculpar*

accused: *procesado*

accustom (v.): *habituar*

ace: *as*

ache (v.): *doler*

ache: *achaque*

ache; back: *dolor de espalda*

ache; belly: *dolor de barriga*

ache; head: *dolor de cabeza*

ache; heart: *angustia*

ache; stomach: *dolor de estómago, cólicos*

ache; tooth: *dolor de muela, dolor de dientes*

achieve (v.): *lograr, realizar*

achievement: *logro*

acidity: *acedía, acidez*

acidosis: *acidosis*

acquire (v.): *adquirir*

acrobat: *equilibrista, saltimbanqui*

acromegaly: *acromegalía*

act (v.): *actuar*

act: *acto, manejarse*

action: *acción, acto*

activate (v.): *activar*

active: *activo*

activism: *activismo*

activity: *actividad*

actor: *actor, comediante*

actress: *actriz*

acute: *agudo*

adage: *adagio*

adam's apple: *la nuez de adam (adan)*

adapt (v.): *adaptar, aceduar, apropiar*
adaptation: *adaptación*
add (v.): *adicionar*
add up (v.): *sumar*
addict: *adicto*
addicted (to): *adicto (a)*
addiction: *adicción*
additional: *adicional*
additive: *aditivo*
address: *dirección*
adduce (v.): *aducir*
adequate: *adecuado*
adhesive: *pegajoso*
adjacent: *adyacente*
adjective: *adjetivo*
adjoin (v.): *colindar*
adjoining: *lindante*
adjust (v.): *ajustar, acomodar*
adjustment: *ajuste*
administration: *administración*
admirable: *admirable*
admiral: *almirante*
admiration: *admiración*
admire (v.): *admirer*
admission form: *formulario de admisión*
admission: *admisión*
admissions office: *oficina de admisión*
admit; to the hosp. (v.): *ingresar*
adobe: *adobe*
adolescence: *adolescencía*
adopt (v.): *adoptar, prohijar*
adoption: *adopción*
adore (v.): *adorar*
adrenaline: *adrenalina*
adult: *adulto, mayor de edad*
adultery: *adulterio*
advance: *adelantamiento*
advanced: *adelantado*
advantage: *provecho, ventaja*
adventure: *aventura*
adverb: *adverbio*
adversary: *adversario*
adverse: *adverso*
advice: *consejo*
advise (v.): *aconsejar*
aerial: *aéreo*
affability: *agrado*
affable: *afable*
affair: *cosa*
affect (v.): *afectar*
affectation: *afectación*
affection: *afección*

affinity: *afinidad*
affirm (v.): *afirmar*
affirmative: *afirmativo*
afflict (v.): *afligir*
affront: *afrenta*
africa: *africa*
african: *africano*
after: *después (de)*
afternoon: *(la) tarde*
aftertaste: *despues de probar, regusto*
again: *nuevamente, otra vez*
against: *contra*
age: *edad*
aged: *anciano*
agency: *agencia*
agenda: *orden del día, agenda*
agent: *agente*
aggravate (v.): *agravar*
aggressive: *agresivo, agresión*
agile: *ágil*
agility: *agilidad*
ago: *"hace" + reference of time, e.g. "2 days ago" is "hace dos días"*
agrarian: *agrario*
agree with: *estar de acuerdo con*
agreeable: *agradable*
agreed: *de acuerdo*
ahead: *adelante*
ailing: *enfermo*
ailment: *malestar*
aim: *puntería*
air conditioning: *aire acondicionado*
air: *aire*
air; by air: *por vía aérea*
airplane: *avion*
airport: *aeropuerto*
airsick: *mareado en el aire*
aisle: *pasillo, nave*
alarm: *alarma*
alas: *"¡ay!", "¡ay de mí!"*
albania: *albania*
alberian: *argelino*
albinism: *albinismo*
album: *álbum*
alchemy: *alquimia*
alcohol: *alcohol*
alcoholic: *alcohólico*
alcoholism: *alcoholismo*
alder: *aliso*
ale: *ale, cerveza inglesa*
alert: *alerta, despabilado*
algebra: *álgebra*
algeria: *argelia*
alias: *alias*

alibi: *exucsa, coartada*
alienate (v.): *alienar, enajenar*
alienation: *alienación*
align (v.): *alinear*
alike: *igualmente, parecido, semejantes*
alimentation: *alimentación*
alimony: *alimentos*
alive: *vivo*
alkalosis: *alcalosis*
all over: *por todo*
all that: *cuanto*
all-purpose: *para todo uso*
all-weather: *para todo tiempo*
all: *todo(s)*
allege (v.): *alegar*
allergic reaction: *reaccion alérgica*
allergic: *alérgico*
allergy: *alergía*
alley: *callejuela, calleja*
alliance: *alianza*
allied: *aliado*
alligator: *caimán*
alloy: *aleación*
allude: *aludir a*
allusion: *alusión*
allusive: *alusivo*
alluvium: *aluvión*
ally (v.): *aliar*
almanac: *almanaque*
almond: *almendra*
almost: *casi*
alone: *solo*
aloud: *en voz alta, alto*
alphabet: *abecedario, alfabeto*
already: *ya*
also: *también*
alter (v.): *alterar, inmutar*
alteration: *alteración*
alternate (v.): *alternar*
alternative: *alternativa*
although: *aunque*
altitude: *altitud*
altogether: *enteramente, en conjunto*
altruism: *altruismo*
aluminum: *aluminio*
always: *siempre*
amalgam: *amalgama*
amateur: *amateur*
amaze (v.): *asombrar*
ambassador: *embajador*
amber: *ámbar*
ambiguous: *ambiguo, promiscuo*
ambitious: *ambicioso*

ambulance: *ambulancía*
ambulant: *ambulante*
ambulatory: *ambulatorio*
ambush: *celada*
amen: *amén*
amenity: *amenidad*
america: *américa*
amethyst: *amatista*
amiability: *amabilidad*
amiable: *amable*
amid: *en medio de*
amnesia: *pérdida de memoria "loss of memory", amnesia*
amnesty: *amnistía*
amoeba: *amiba*
amoebiasis: *amebiasis*
among: *entre*
amorous: *amoroso-a*
amount: *cauntidad*
amphetamine: *anfetamina*
amplification: *amplificación*
amplifier: *amplificador*
amplify (v.): *amplicar*
amputate (v.): *amputar*
amuse (v.): *solazar*
amusing: *chistoso, distraído*
anachronism: *anacronismo*
anaemia: *anemia*
analgesic: *analgésico*
analgesía: *analgesía*
analogy: *analogía*
analysis: *análisis*
analytic: *analítico*
analyze (v.): *analizar*
anaphylactic: *anafiláctico*
anarchy: *anarquía*
anatomy: *anatomía*
ancestor: *progenitor*
ancestors: *antepasados*
ancestry: *abolengo*
anchor: *anclar*
anchovy: *anchoa*
ancient: *antiguo*
and so: *conque*
and: *y*
andorra: *andorra*
anecdote: *anécdota*
anemia: *anemía*
anesthesia: *anestesia*
anesthesia; caudal: *anestesia caudal*
anesthesia; general: *anestesia general*
anesthesia; local: *anestesia local*
anesthesiologist: *anestesiólogo-a*
anesthesiology department:

departamento de anestesiología
anesthesiology: *anestesiología*
anesthetic: *anestético*
anesthetize (v.): *anestesiar*
aneurysm: *aneurisma*
angel: *ángel*
anger (v.): *airar*
angina: *angina*
angle: *ángulo*
anglicism: *anglicismo*
angry: *airado, colérico, enojado*
anguish: *angustia, congoja, traspaso*
animal: *animal*
animate (v.): *animar*
animated: *animado*
animosity: *animosidad*
aniseed: *anís*
ankle: *tobillo*
annals: *anales*
annex (v.): *anexar*
anniversary: *aniversario*
announce: *anunciación*
annoy (v.): *desazonar*
annoy: *enojado-a*
annual: *anual*
annul (v.): *anular*
anomaly: *anomalía*
anonymous: *anónimo*
anorexia: *anorexía*
another: *otro*
answer (v.): *contestar*
ant: *hormiga*
antacid: *antiácido*
antelope: *antílope*
antenna: *antena*
anteroom: *antesala*
antibiotic: *antibiótico*
anticipate (v.): *anticipar*
antidote: *antídoto*
antifreeze: *anticongelante*
antihistamine: *antihistamina*
antipathy: *antipatía*
antique: *antigualla*
antiquity: *antigüedad*
antiseptic: *antiséptico*
antispasmodic: *antiespasmódico*
antitetanic: *antitetánico*
anuresis: *anuresis*
anuria: *anuría*
anus: *ano*
anxiety: *ansiedad, ansia*
anxious: *ansioso*
any: *alguno, cualquier*
anything: *algo*

anyway: *de todas maneras*
aortic: *aórtico*
apartment: *apartamento*
apathy: *apatía*
aplomb: *aplomo*
apologize (v.): *excusar*
apologize: *disculparse, excusarse*
apostle: *apóstol*
apostrophe: *apóstrofo*
apparent: *aparente*
apparition: *aparicion, estanigua, fantasma*
appear (v.): *comparecer, presentar*
appearance: *apariencia, aspecto*
appendicitis: *apendicitis*
appendix: *apéndice*
appetite: *apetito*
appitcable: *aplicable*
applaud (v.): *aplaudir, palmotear*
apple tree: *manzano*
apple: *manzana*
appliance: *aparato*
applicant: *solicitante*
application: *aplicación*
apply (v.): *aplicar*
apply; to oneself: *aplicarse*
appoint (v.): *adscribir*
appointment: *cita*
appraise (v.): *avaluar*
appreciate (v.): *apreciar*
apprehension: *aprensión*
apprentice: *aprendiz*
approach (v.): *acercar a, abocar*
approach: *acercarse a, abocarse*
appropriate: *apropiado*
approval: *aprobación*
approve (v.): *aprobar*
approximation: *aproximación*
apricot: *albaricoque*
april: *abril*
apron: *delantal, mandil*
aptitude: *aptitud*
aquarium: *acuario*
aquatic: *acuático*
arab: *árabe*
arable: *labrantío*
arbitrate (v.): *arbitrar*
arcade: *arcada*
arch; arc: *arco*
archaic: *arcaico*
archer: *arquero*
arching: *arqueo*
architect: *arquitecto*
archive: *archivo*

arctic: *ártico*
arduous: *arduo*
are there; is there: *¿hay...?*
area: *área, zona*
arena: *arena*
argentina: *argentina*
argue (v.): *argumentar*
argument: *altercado, argumentación, argumento*
aria: *aria*
arid: *árido*
aridity: *aridez*
arise (v.): *surgir*
arm; attached to shoulder: *brazo*
arm; with weapons: *arma*
armchair: *butaca, sillón*
armed: *armado*
armful: *brazada*
armor: *armadura*
armpit: *axila, sobaco*
army: *ejército*
aroma: *aroma*
around: *alrededor*
arouse (v.): *apasionar*
arrange (v.): *arreglar, acondicionar*
arrangement: *acomodo*
array (v.): *ataviar*
arrears: *atrasos*
arrest (v.): *arrestar*
arrested: *detenido*
arrhythmia: *arritmia*
arrival: *advenimiento, llegada*
arrive (v.): *llegar*
arrogance: *arrogancía*
arrogant: *arrogante*
arrow: *flecha, saeta*
arsenal: *aresenal*
arsenic: *arsénico*
art: *arte*
arteriogram: *arteriograma*
arteriosclerosis: *arterioesclerosis*
artery: *arteria*
arthritis: *artritis*
artichoke: *alcachofa*
article: *artículo*
articulate (v.): *articular*
articulation: *articulación*
artificial respiration: *respiración artificial*
artificial: *artificial*
artisan: *artesano, artífice*
artist: *artista*
as for: *en cuanto a*
as much: *tanto*

as soon as possible: *cuanto antes, lo más pronto posible*
as soon as: *tan pronto como*
as: *tan, como*
asbestos: *asbesto*
ascend (v.): *ascender*
asceticism: *ascetismo*
ash: *ceniza*
ashtray: *cenicero*
asia: *asia*
asian: *asiático*
asiatic: *asiático*
ask (v.): *preguntar, requerir*
ask a question: *hacer una pregunta*
ask for (v.): *solicitar, pedir*
asleep: *dormido*
asp: *áspid*
asparagus: *espárrago*
aspect: *aspecto*
asphalt: *asfalto*
aspiration: *aspiracion, pretensión*
aspirin: *aspirina*
assault (v.): *asaltar*
assembly: *asamblea*
assent (v.): *asentir*
assiduous: *asiduo*
assign (v.): *asignar*
assigned: *asignado*
assignment: *asignación*
assimilation: *asimilacion*
assist (v.): *asistir*
assistance: *auxilio, ayuda, asistencía*
assistant: *ayudante, asistente*
association: *asociación, asociado*
assume (v.): *asumir*
assumption: *asunción*
assure (v.): *asegurar*
asthenia: *astenía*
asthma: *asma*
astigmatism: *astigmatismo*
astrology: *astrología*
astutue: *astuto*
asylum: *asilo*
at (time): *a las*
at least: *por lo menos*
at noon: *al mediodía*
at once: *en este momento*
at that time: *a esta hora, entonces*
at the house of: *en casa de*
at the same time: *al mismo tiempo*
at the side of: *al lado de*
at times: *a veces*
at: *a, en*
atherosclerosis: *ateroesclerosis,*

arteroesclerosis
athlete: *atleta*
atlas: *atlas*
atmosphere: *ambiente, atmosfera*
atom: *átomo*
atomic: *átomico*
atomizer: *atomizador*
atrocious: *atroz*
atrocity: *atrocidad*
atrophy: *atrofía*
attach (v.): *adjuntar*
attachment: *apego*
attack (v.): *acometer, atacar*
attack: *acometerse, ataque*
attempt (v.): *atentar*
attempt suicide (v.): *atentar el suicidio*
attendant: *asistente-a*
attention: *atención*
attentive: *atento, attenuate*
attic: *ático, desván, guardilla*
attire: *atavío*
attitude: *actitud, postura*
attorney: *abogado*
attract (v.): *atraer*
attraction: *atracción*
attractive: *atractivo-a*
auction: *almoneda*
audience: *asistencia, audiencia*
auditor: *auditor*
august: *agosto*
aunt: *tía*
austere: *austero*
austria: *austria*
author: *autor, autora*
authority: *autoridad*
authorization: *autorización*
authorize (v.): *autorizar, apoderar*
autograph: *autógrafo*
automatic: *automático*
automobile: *auto, automóvil*
autopsy: *autopsía*
autumn (fall): *ontoño*
available: *disponible*
avalanche: *alud, avalancha*
avarice: *avaricia*
avenue: *avenida*
average: *medio*
average; mean: *promedio*
aviation: *aviación*
aviator (pilot): *aviador*
avid: *ávido*
avidity: *avidez*
avitaminosis: *avitaminosis*

avoid (v.): *eludir, evitar*
awake: *despierto*
awaken (v.): *despertar*
awaken: *despertarse*
aware of: *enterado-a*
away from: *lejos de*
axe: *hacha, segur*
axiom: *axioma*
axis: *aje*
aztec: *azteca*

B

b.i.d.; twice a day: *dos veces por día*
b.p. cuff: *baumanómetro*
baby teeth: *dientes de leche "milk teeth"*
baby-sitter: *niñera, niñeratomada por horas*
baby: *nene, nena, niño, niña, bebé*
bachelor: *soltero, mancebo*
back ; behind: *atras, envés*
back ; low spine: *espalda*
back of the hand: *dorso de la mano*
backache: *dolor de espalda*
backbone: *espina dorsal, espinazo*
backward; primitive: *regresivo*
backwards: *atrás*
bacon: *tocino*
bacteriology: *bacteriología*
bad taste: *mal sabor*
bad: *malo, mala, mal*
badly: *mal*
baffle (v.): *desconcertar*
bag: *bolsa, maletín, saco*
bag; hot water: *bolsa de agua caliente*
bag; ice: *bolsa de hielo*
bag; water: *bolsa de agua*
baggage: *equipaje, bagaje*
bail: *caución*
baked potato: *papa asada*
baked: *al horno*
baker: *panadero*
bakery: *panadería*
balance (v.): *abalanzar, balancear*
balanced: *balanceado*
balcony: *balcón, terraza*
bald spot: *calvo*
bald: *calvo, calva*
baldness: *calvicie*
ball: *balón*
ballad: *cantinela, romance*
ballast: *lastre*

ballet: *ballet*
ballplayer: *pelotero*
ballpoint pen: *bolígrafo, picera*
bamboo: *bambú*
banana: *banana, plátano*
band-aid®: *curita*
band: *cinta*
bandage: *venda*
bandage; elastic: *venda elástica*
bandit: *bandido*
bank: *bancario, banco*
bank; blood: *banco de sangre*
banker: *banquero*
bankrupt: *bancarrota*
banquet: *banquete*
baptism: *bautismo*
baptist: *bautista*
baptize (v.): *bautizar*
bar (v.): *atrancar*
barbaric: *barbarico*
barbecue: *barbacoa*
barber: *peluquero, barbero*
barbiturate: *barbiturato, barbitúrico*
bargain: *avenencia, chollo*
barge: *barcaza*
barium sulfate: *sulfato de bario*
bark: *corteza*
barking: *ladrido*
barley: *cebada*
barman: *barman*
barmy: *guillado*
barometer: *barómetro*
baroque: *barroco*
barrel: *barril*
barrier: *barrera*
bartender: *cantinero, tabernero*
base: *base*
basement: *sótano*
baseness: *bajeza*
basic: *básico*
basin: *bacin, basía*
basket: *canasta, cesta*
basque: *éuscaro*
bass drum: *bombo*
bassinette: *cunita/el moisés/bacinete*
bastard: *bastardo*
bastion: *baluarte*
bat: *bate*
bath: *baño*
bathe (v.): *bañar*
bathe onself: *bañarse*
bather: *bañista*
bathing: *malla*
bathrobe: *bata*

bathroom, public restroom: *los servicios públicos, los servicios sanitarios*
bathroom: *baño, cuarto de baño, "wc", excusado, servicio*
bathtub; for adults: *tina*
bathtub; for the baby: *el bacín (para el niño)*
baton: *batuta*
batter: *bateador*
battery: *batería, pila*
battle: *batalla, pugna*
bay: *bahía*
bayonet: *bayoneta*
bazaar: *bazar*
be (passive voice) (v.): *ser*
be (v.): *estar; ser*
be able (v.): *poder*
be ashamed (v.): *afrentar*
be bored (v.): *aburrir*
be born (v.): *nacer*
be called (v.): *llamar*
be cold (v.): *tener frio*
be dizzy (v.): *tener mareo, estar mareado*
be hot (v.): *tener calor*
be hungry (v.): *tener hambre*
be injured (v.): *lesionar*
be interested in (v.): *estar interesado en*
be named (v.): *llamar*
be poisoned (v.): *envenenar*
be right (v.): *tener razón*
be to (v.): *haber de*
beach: *playa*
beacon: *baliza*
beak: *pico*
beam: *madero, tablón*
bean: *habichuela, frijoles, haba*
bear (v.): *aguantar*
bear; animal: *oso*
bear; to give birth: *parir, dar a luz*
beard: *barba*
bearded: *barbado, barbudo*
beat it; get away: *largarse*
beat; hit (v.): *apalear, azotar*
beaten: *batido*
beating: *aporreo, paliza*
beautiful: *bello-a, hermoso*
beauty: *beldad, belleza, hermosura*
beaver: *castor*
because of: *a causa de*
because: *porque*
become (v.): *ponerse, cansarse*

become blurred: *ponerse borroso*
become pregnant: *embarazarse*
become sick: *enfermarse*
bed linen: *ropa de cama*
bed: *cama*
bedbug: *chinche*
bedpan (slang): *comodo, cuna (slang), paleta, silleta (bedside commode), taza*
bedpan: *el bacin*
bedroom: *alcoba*
bedside commode: *silleta*
bedspread: *cobertor*
bee: *abeja*
beef: *carne de vaca, carne de res*
beefsteak: *bistec*
beehive: *colmena*
beer: *cerveza*
beet: *remolecha*
beetle: *escarabajo*
before: *antes (de)*
beg (v.): *mendigar*
beggar: *mendigo, pordiosero*
begin (v.): *comenzar, empezar*
beginner: *novel*
beginning: *comienzo, principio*
behave (v.): *comportar*
behave oneself: *comportarse*
behavior: *comportamiento*
behead (v.): *descabezar*
behind: *atrás, detrás de, tras*
belch (v.): *eructar, tener eructos, repetir*
belch: *eructo, repete, regüeldo*
belgium: *bélgica*
belief: *creencia*
believe (v.): *creer, pensar*
believer: *creyente*
bell: *timbre, campana*
bellow (v.): *berrear, bramar*
belly ache: *dolor de barriga*
belly: *panza, barriga*
belong (v.): *pertenecer*
beloved: *amado*
below: *abajo*
belt: *cinto, cinturón*
bench: *banca*
bend (v.): *agachar, doblar*
bend down: *bajarse*
bend: *doble*
beneficial: *beneficioso*
benefit (v.): *beneficiar*
bent: *cacho*
beret: *biona*

berth: *litera*
beside: *tras de*
besides: *además (de)*
best: *emejor*
bestial: *bestial*
bet (v.): *apostar*
better: *mejor*
between: *entre*
bewildered: *atontado, embabado*
beyond: *más allá de*
bib: *babero*
bible: *biblia*
bibliography: *bibliografí*
bicuspid: *bicúspide*
bicycle: *bicicleta*
bidet: *bidé*
biennial: *bienal*
bifocals: *bifocales*
big wave: *oleada*
big: *grande*
bigamy: *bigamia*
bile duct: *conducto biliar*
bile: *hiel, bilis*
bilingual: *bilingüe*
bill (restaurant): *cuenta, factura*
billiards: *billar*
billion: *billón*
bind (v.): *astringir*
binoculars: *prismáticos*
biology: *biología*
biopsy: *biopsía*
biplane: *biplano*
birch: *abedul*
bird: *ave, pájaro*
birth control method: *método anti-conceptivo*
birth: *nacimiento, natalidad*
birthmark: *marca de nacimiento, lunar, mancha mongolica*
births; multiple: *parto múltiple*
births; natural: *parto natural*
births; premature: *parto prematuro*
biscuit: *bizcocho, galleta*
bison: *bisonte*
bite: *morder, mordisco*
bite; bee (sting): *picadura de abejas*
bite; cat: *mordedura de gato*
bite; dog: *mordedura de perro*
bite; flea: *picadura de pulga*
bite; human: *mordedura de persona*
bite; mosquito: *mordedura de mollote, mordedura de mosquito*
bite; of an insect: *picadura*
bite; scorpion (sting): *picadura de*

elalacran
bite; snake: *mordedura de culebra*
bite; spider (sting): *picadura de araña*
biting: *mordaz*
bitter: *agrio, amargo, acerbo, acre*
bitterness: *amargura*
black: *negro*
blackberry: *zarzamora*
blackbird: *mirlo*
blackboard: *tablero*
blackness: *negrura*
blackout: *vision negra, apagón*
blacksmith: *herrero*
bladder: *vejiga*
blade: *cuchilla*
bland: *blando, suave*
blanket: *cobija, frazada, manta*
blankets: *cobijitas*
bleach: *blanqueador*
bleed (v.): *desangrar, sangrar*
bleeding disorder: *enfermedades hemorrágicas*
bleeding tendency: *tendencia a sangrar*
bleeding: *sangrado*
blind: *ciego*
blindness: *ceguera*
blink (v.): *parpadear*
blister: *vejiga, ampolla*
blonde: *rubio*
blood bank: *banco de sangre*
blood count: *conteo globular*
blood gas: *prueba de sangre arterial*
blood pressure: *presión arterial, presión sanguínea*
blood pressure; cuff: *baumanómetro*
blood pressure; high: *presion alta*
blood pressure; low: *presión baja*
blood test: *prueba de sangre*
blood: *sangre*
blow; breathe (v.): *soplar*
blow; to strike: *golpe*
blow; with lungs: *sopla*
blue: *azul*
blurred: *borroso*
blushing; flushing: *bochornos*
board (v.): *entablar*
board: *tabla*
boarding: *pensión*
boast: *bravata*
boat: *barca, bote, barco*
boatman: *barquero*
body: *armazón, cuerpo*
bog: *canagal*

bohemian: *bohemio*
boil (v.): *bullir*
boil: *bullirse, divieso*
boiled: *hervido*
boiler: *caldera*
boiling: *ebullición, hirviente*
bold: *audaz*
boldness: *audacia*
bolivia: *bolivia*
bomb: *bomba*
bomber: *bombardero*
bond: *atadura*
bones: *huesos*
bonnet: *capota*
bonus: *bonus, plus*
bony: *óseo, huesudo*
book seller: *librero*
book: *libro*
bookkeeper: *tenedor de libros*
bookstore: *librería*
boom: *auge*
boot: *bota, portaequipajes, portamaletas*
booth: *cabina*
booty: *botín*
border: *bordear*
bordering: *afín*
bore (v.): *aburrir*
bored: *aburrido*
borer: *barreno*
boring: *tedioso*
born in: *nacido en, nacida en*
born: *nacido*
boss: *jefe, patrón*
both: *ambos, los dos*
bother (v.): *molestar*
bother: *estorbo, molestia*
bothersome: *molesto*
bottle (v.): *embotellar*
bottle: *botella, frasco*
bottle; baby's: *biberon*
bottle; nipple: *pezón de biberón*
bottom; at bottom: *en el fondo*
bottom; of jar: *culo*
bottom; price: *más bajo*
bottom; rectum; anus: *ano*
bottom; to go to the bottom (v.): *irse a pique*
botulism: *botulismo*
boulder: *canto rodado*
bounce: *bote*
bowel movement (v.): *obrar*
bowels: *intestinos*
bowl: *bola, tazón*

bowlegged: *corvo*
bowman: *arquero*
box up (v.): *encajonar*
box: *arca, estuche*
boxer: *boxeador*
boxing: *boxeo*
boy: *muchacho, zagal*
boycott (v.): *boicotear*
boycott: *boicotearse, biocoteo*
boyfriend: *novio*
bra: *sostén*
brace: *braguero*
bracelet: *ajorca, brazalete, pulsera*
brag (v.): *blasonar*
brain: *cerebro*
brave: *valiente*
bread: *pan*
bread; rye: *pan de centeno*
bread; sweet bread: *pan dulce*
bread; white: *pan blanco*
bread; whole wheat: *pan de trigo entero*
break (v.): *quebrar, romper*
breakfast: *desayuno*
breast cancer: *cáncer de los pechos*
breast feed (v.): *dar el pecho, mamar*
breastbone: *esternón*
breasts: *senos, pechos*
breathe (v.): *respirar*
bridge: *puente*
brilliant: *brillante*
bring (v.): *traer*
broccoli: *brócoli*
broiled: *a la parrilla*
broke: *arruinado-a*
broken: *quebrado, quebrada*
bronchi: *bronquios*
bronchial tubes: *bronquios*
bronchitis: *bronquitis*
bronchopneumonia: *bronconeumonía*
brother-in-law: *cuñado*
brother: *hermano*
brown: *cafe, marrón*
brucellosis: *brucelosis*
bruise: *moretón, contusión*
brun: *quemadura*
brunette: *moreno*
brush (v.): *cepillar*
brush: *cepillo*
brush; hair: *cepillo para el cabello*
brush; tooth: *cepillo para el dientes*
bubble (v.): *burbojear*
bubble: *burbuja, pompa*

bubonic: *bubónico*
bucket: *balde*
buckle: *hebilla*
budget: *presupuesto*
buffalo: *búfalo*
buffet: *fonda*
bug: *bicho*
bugle: *clarín*
builder: *constructor*
building: *edificio*
bulb: *bombilla*
bulky: *abultado*
bull: *bula, toro*
bullet wound: *balazo*
bullet: *bala*
bulletin: *boletín*
bullfight: *lidia*
bully: *matón*
bump into (v.): *topar*
bump: *bulto, protuberancia, chichón*
bumper: *parachoques, paragolpes*
bun: *moño*
bunch: *gajo*
bundle: *lío*
buoy: *boya*
burden: *gravamen*
bureaucracy: *burocracia*
burglar: *ganzúa*
burn (v.): *quemar, abrasar*
burn oneself: *quemarse*
burning: *ardiente, quemante*
burnous: *albornoz*
bursitis: *bursitis*
bury (v.): *enterrar*
bus: *autobús*
bush: *arbusto*
business: *negocio*
businessman: *comerciante, hombre de negocios*
bust: *busto*
bustle: *ajetreo*
busy: *atareado, ocupado*
but: *pero, mas*
butane: *butano*
butcher's shop: *carnicería*
butcher: *carnicero*
butler: *mayordomo*
butter: *mantequilla*
butterfly: *mariposa*
buttocks: *nalgas*
button (v.): *abotonar*
button: *botón*
buyer: *comprador*
buzz: *rumor*

buzzer: *zumbador*

C

cabaret: *cabaret*
cabbage: *berza, col, repollo*
cabinet: *gabinete*
cable: *cable*
cablegram: *cablegrama*
cactus: *cacto*
cadence: *cadencia*
caesarean section: *sección cesarea*
cafeteria: *cafetería, cafetín*
cage: *jaula*
cake: *torta, tarta, pastel, pastilla*
calamine: *calamina*
calamity: *calamidad*
calcification: *calcificación*
calcium: *calcio*
calculate (v.): *calcular*
calculation: *cálculo, tanteo*
calendar: *calendario*
calf: *pantorrilla, ternero*
call (v.): *llamar*
callus: *callo*
calm (v.): *calmar*
calm oneself: *calmarse, aplacarse, serenarse*
calm: *tranquilo, calma*
calorie: *caloría*
calvary: *calvario*
calves: *pantorrillas*
camel: *camello*
camomile: *manzanilla*
camp (v.): *acampar*
campaign: *campaña*
camping: *camping*
can (v.): *poder*
canada: *canadá*
canal: *canal*
canary: *canario*
cancel (v.): *cancelar*
cancellation: *cancelación*
cancer: *cáncer*
cancerous: *canceroso*
candidiasis: *moniliasis*
candle: *vela*
candy store: *confitería*
candy; sweets: *dulces, bombóm*
cane: *bastón*
canine: *canino*
canker sores: *postemilla*
canoe: *canoa, piragua*

canon: *canónigo*
canteen: *cantimplora, cantina*
canteloupe: *cantalup*
canvas: *lienzo*
cap: *gorro*
capable: *capaz, susceptible de*
capacity: *capacidad*
caper: *cabriola*
capital: *capital*
capsule: *cápsula*
captain: *capitán*
captive: *cautivo*
capture: *captura*
car seat; for infant: *asiento para carro, asiento de seguridad*
car: *automóvil, auto*
carafe: *garrafa*
carat: *quilate*
caravan: *caravana*
carbine: *carabina*
carbon: *carbono*
carbon paper: *papel carbón*
card: *tarjeta*
cardboard: *cartón*
cardiac: *cardíaco*
cardinal: *cardenal*
cardiologist: *cardiólogo*
cardiology: *cardiología*
cards: *naipes*
care (for) (v.): *cuidar (a)*
care: *cuidado*
careful: *cauteloso*
carefully: *con cuidado, cuidadosamente*
careless: *sin cuidado, dejado, descuidado*
caress (v.): *acariciar*
carnal: *carnal*
carnation: *clavel*
carnival: *carnaval*
carnivorous: *carnivoro*
carpenter: *carpintero*
carpet (v.): *alfombrar*
carpet: *alfombra, tapiz*
carrier; of disease: *portador de enfermedad*
carrot: *zanahoria*
carry (v.): *llevar*
carry on a stretcher (v.): *llevar en camilla*
carry out (v.): *cumplir*
cart: *carro*
case; bag: *caja*
case; in case: *caso*

cash (v.): *cobrar*
cashier; office: *caja*
cashier; person: *cajero*
cask: *cuba*
cast: *yeso*
caste: *casta*
castle: *castillo*
castrate (v.): *capar*
cat: *gato*
cataracts: *cataratas*
catch (v.): *cachar*
catch a disease (v.): *contraer una enfermedad*
catch cold (v.): *resfriar*
catch: *cogerse*
catch; catch cold: *refriarse*
catch; catch fire: *encenderse*
catch; of a ball: *cogida*
category: *categoría*
caterpillar: *oruga*
cathedral: *catedral*
catheter: *catéter, sonda*
catholic: *católico*
catholicism: *catolicismo*
catsup: *salsa de tomate*
cattleman: *ganadero*
cauliflower: *coliflor*
cause (v.): *causar*
cause: *causa*
caustic: *cáustico*
cauterizatlon: *cauterización*
caution: *cautela*
cautious: *prudente, cauto*
cave: *cueva*
cavern: *antro, canverna*
cavity: *carie, cavidad*
cease (v.): *cesar*
cedar: *cedro*
celebrate (v.): *celebrar*
celebration: *celebración*
celery: *apio*
celibacy: *celibato*
celibate: *célibe*
cell: *celda*
cellar: *bodega*
cement (v.): *cementar*
cemetery: *campo santo, cemeterio, pateon*
censor: *censor*
censure (v.): *censurar*
censure: *censura*
census: *censo*
center: *centro*
centigrade: *centígrado*

central: *central*
century: *siglo*
ceramic: *cerámico*
cereal: *cereal*
cerebral palsy: *parálisis cerebral*
certain: *cierto*
certificate: *acta, cédula, certificado*
certification: *certificación*
certify (v.): *certificar*
cerumen; earwax: *cera, cerilla*
cervical cap: *gorro cervical*
cervix: *cerviz, cuello uterino, cuello de la matriz*
cessation: *cesación*
chain (v.) : *encadenar*
chain: *cadena*
chair: *silla*
chalk: *gis, tiza*
challenge (v.): *desafiar*
chamber: *cámara*
chamois: *gamuza*
champion: *campeón*
chance (v.): *azar*
chancre: *chancro*
change (v.): *cambiar*
change of life: *cambio de vida*
change: *cambio, cambiarse*
channel (v.): *canalizar*
chaos: *caos*
chapel: *capilla*
chapter: *cabildo, capítulo*
character: *carácter*
characteristic: *característico*
charge: *carga, encomienda*
charity: *beneficencia, caridad*
charm: *donaire, talisman*
chart (record): *ficha, historia personal, fila*
chase (v.): *cazar*
chassis: *armazón*
chaste: *casto*
chat (v.): *charlar*
chatter: *garrulería*
chauffeur: *chofer, chófer*
cheap: *barato, barata*
cheat: *petardista*
chechoslovakia: *checoslovaquia*
check: *comprobar, cheque, chequeo*
checkup: *chequeo, chequeo médico*
cheek: *cachete, mejilla, carrillo*
cheep (v.): *piar*
cheer up (v.): *alegrar, refocilar*
cheer up: *alegrarse, animarse*
cheese: *queso*

chemical: *químico*
chemistry: *química*
cherry: *cereza*
chess: *ajedrez*
chest pain: *dolor en el pecho*
chest x-ray: *rayos equis del pecho*
chest: *pecho, tórax*
chest; anatomy: *pecho*
chest; used for storage: *arca*
chew (v.): *masticar, mascar*
chewable: *masticable*
chicken pox: *viruelas locas, vericela*
chicken raiser: *gallinero*
chicken: *pollo*
child abuse: *maltrato de los niños*
child-boy: *niño*
child-girl: *niña*
child: *niño, niña*
childbirth: *parto*
childhood: *niñez*
children: *los niños*
chile: *chile*
chili: *ají, chile*
chills: *calosfrio, escalofríos*
chimney: *chimenea*
chin: *barbilla, mentón, barba*
chips; potato: *papas fritas, patatas fritas*
chiropractor: *quiropractieo, quiropráctor*
chit-chat: *charla, palíque*
chlamydia: *clamidia*
chlorosis: *clorosis*
chocolate: *chocolate*
choice: *escober, escogimiento*
choke (v.): *atragantar*
choke: *estrangulación*
cholesterol: *colesterina, colesterol*
choose (v.): *escoger, elegir*
chop: *chuleta*
chorea: *corea*
chorus: *coro*
chosen: *escogido*
christ: *cristo*
christian name: *nombre de pila*
christian: *cristiano*
christmas eve: *nochebuena*
christmas gift: *regalo de navidad*
christmas tree: *árbol de navidad*
christmas: *navidad*
chrome: *cromo*
chronic disease: *enfermedad crónica*
chronic: *crónico*
church: *iglesia*

churn: *mantequera*
cider: *sidra*
cigar: *cigarro*
cigarette: *cigarrillo, pitillo*
cinema: *cine*
cinnamon: *canela*
circle: *círculo*
circuit: *circuito*
circulate (v.): *circular*
circulation: *circulación*
circulatory: *circulatorio*
circulatory system: *sistema circulatorio*
circumcise (v.): *circuncidar*
circus: *circo*
cirrhosis: *cirrosis*
cistern: *aljibe*
citizen: *ciudadano*
citizenry: *ciudadanía*
citrus fruits: *frutas citricos*
city: *ciudad*
city hall: *municipalidad*
civic: *cívico*
civil: *civil*
civilization: *civilización*
claim: *reclamación*
clam: *almeja*
clamor: *clamoreo*
clap (v.): *batir palmas, palmear*
clarinet: *clarinete*
clarity: *claridad, nitidez*
class: *clase*
classical: *clásico*
classification: *clasificación*
classify (v.): *clasificar*
classroom: *aula*
clause: *cláusula*
clavicle: *clavícula, cuenca, hueso del cuello "neck bone"*
claw: *garfa, garra*
clay: *ancilla*
clean (v.): *limpiar*
clean: *limpio, aseado*
cleaning: *limpieza*
cleanliness: *aseo*
clear away (v.): *obviar*
clear: *claro*
clear up (v.): *aclarar*
clef: *clave*
clemency: *clemencía*
clergy: *pastor, clérigo, clero*
clerk: *dependiente, actuario, oficinista*
clever: *hábil, inteligente*
click: *chasquido*

client: *cliente*
cliff: *despeñadero*
climate: *clima*
climb (v.): *escalar*
clinic: *clínica, clínico*
clinic; dental: *clínica dental*
clinic; outpatient: *clínica paciente-ambulante*
clique: *camarilla*
cloak: *capa, manto*
clock: *reloj*
clog up (v.): *atascar*
clog: *zueco*
close (v.): *cerrar*
close: *allegado, cercano*
closed: *cerrado*
cloth: *paño*
clothes: *ropa*
clothing: *ropa*
cloud (v.): *anublar*
cloud: *nube*
cloud; brain: *nube de cerebro*
cloudy: *nublado*
clown: *payaso*
club: *casino, club*
clumsy: *inhábil*
coach: *autocar*
coagulate (v.): *coagular*
coagulation: *coagulación*
coal: *brasa, carbón*
coarse: *curro*
coast: *costa, litoral*
coat: *abrigo*
cobra: *cobra*
cocaine: *cocaina*
coccyx: *colita, coxis*
cockroach: *cucaracha*
cocoa: *cacao*
coconut: *coco*
cod: *bacalao*
cod liver oil: *aceite de pescado*
code: *cifrar, código*
codeine: *codeina*
coffee: *café*
coffin: *ataúd*
cohabit (v.): *cohabitar*
coin (v.): *acuñar*
coincidence: *coincidencia*
coitus: *coito*
cold (illness): *frio, catarro, resfriado, gripe*
cold (temperature): *frío*
cold pack: *emplasto frío*
cold sore: *ulceras de la boca "ulcers of the mouth"*
coldness: *frialdad*
colectomy: *colectomía*
colic: *cólico*
colitis: *colitis*
collapse: *colapso*
collar bone: *clavicula*
colleague: *colega*
collect (v.): *colectar*
college: *colegio*
collide (v.): *chocar*
collision: *colisión*
colon: *colon*
colonel: *coronel*
colonize (v.): *colonizar*
colony: *colonia*
color: *color*
colorless: *incoloro*
column: *columna*
coma: *coma*
comb (v.): *peinar*
comb: *peine*
combat: *cambate, lid*
combination: *combinación*
come (v.): *venir, regresar*
come apart: *descoserse*
come from: *provenir de*
come in: *¡pase!*
come off: *desgajarse*
comedy: *comedia*
comet: *cometa*
comfort: *comodidad*
comfortable: *cómodo*
comic: *bufo, cómico*
coming: *venidero*
comma: *coma*
command: *comandancia*
comment: *comentario, glosa*
commentary: *comentario*
commercial: *comercial*
commission: *comisión*
commit: *cometer*
committee: *comité*
common: *común*
commotion: *revuelo*
communicable: *comunicable*
communicate (v.): *comunicar*
communication: *comunicación*
community: *comunidad*
compact: *compacto*
companion: *compañero*
company: *compañía*
comparable: *comparable*
compare (v.): *comparar*

comparison: *comparación*
compartment: *compartimiento*
compassion: *compasión*
compensate (v.): *compensar*
compensatory: *compensatorio*
compete: *competir*
competency: *competencia*
competent: *competente*
compile (v.): *compilar*
complacent: *complaciente*
complain (v.): *quejar*
complain: *queja*
complete: *completa*
complex: *complejo*
complexion: *cutis*
complication: *complicación*
compress: *compresa, aplicaciones*
compress; cold: *compresa frío, aplicaciones frío*
compress; hot: *compresa caliente, aplicaciones calientes*
compress; press down (v.): *comprimir*
compresszon: *compresión*
computer: *computadoras*
comrade: *camarada*
concede (v.): *conceder*
concentrate (v.): *concentrar*
concentration: *concentración*
concept: *concepto*
concern: *preocupación*
concise: *conciso*
conclude (v.): *concluir*
conclusion: *conclusión, terminación*
condemn (v.): *condenar*
condiment: *condimento*
condition: *condición*
condom: *condón, hule, preservativo*
conduct; lead (v.): *conducir*
conductor: *conductor*
condyloma: *condiloma*
cone: *barquillo*
conference: *conferencia*
confess (v.): *confesar*
confess: *condenarse*
confession: *confesión*
confine (v.): *confinar*
confine; in an bed (v.): *confinar en una cama*
confine; in an institution (v.): *confinar en una institución*
confirm (v.): *confirmar, revalidar*
confiscate (v.): *confiscar*
conflict: *conflicto*

confront (v.): *afrontar*
confront (with) (v.): *enfrentar (con)*
confuse (v.): *embrollar, trabucar, trastornar*
confused: *confundido, confuso*
confusion: *confusión*
congestion: *congestión*
congratulate (v.): *felicitar*
congratulations: *felicitaciónes*
congregation: *congregación*
congress: *congreso*
conjugal: *conyugal*
conjunctivitis: *conjuntivitis*
connect (v.): *conectar*
connection: *conexión*
conscience: *conciencia*
conscious: *consciente*
consent: *consentimiento*
consequence: *consecuencia*
conservable: *conservable*
conservation: *conservación*
conserve (v.): *conservar*
consider (v.): *considerar*
considerable: *apreciable, considerable*
consideration: *consideración*
consist (v.): *consistir*
consonant: *consonante*
conspirator: *conspirador*
constable: *alguacil*
constancy: *constancia*
constant: *constante*
constipate (v.): *constipar, estreñir*
constipated: *estreñido*
constipation: *constipación, estreñimiento*
constitution: *constitución*
construction: *construcción*
consul: *cónsul*
consulate: *consulado*
consult (v.): *consultar*
consultation: *consulta*
consulting (office): *consultorio*
consume (v.): *consumir*
consumer: *comsumidor*
contact: *contacto*
contact lens(-es): *lente(s) de contacto*
contagious: *contagioso*
contain (v.): *contener*
contaminate (v.): *contaminar*
contamination: *contaminación*
content: *contento*
continuity: *continuidad*
continuously: *continuamente, seguido*

contraception: *contracepción*
contraceptive: *anticonceptivo*
contract (v.): *contraer*
contraction (of labor): *las dolores (del parto)*
contraction: *contracción, los dolores*
contradict (v.): *contradecir*
contrary: *contrario*
contrast: *contraste*
contribute (v.): *aportar, contribuir, ofrendar*
control (v.): *controlar, intervenir*
control: *control*
controllable: *controlable*
convalencence: *convalescencía*
convalescent: *convaleciente*
convenient: *conveniente*
conventionalism: *convencionalismo*
conversation: *conversación*
converse (v.): *conversar*
convert (v.): *convertir*
convict: *presidiario*
conviction: *convicción*
convince (v.): *decidir*
convulsion: *convulsión*
cook (person): *cocinero*
cook (v.): *cocer, cocinar*
cookie: *gelleta dulce*
cool (v.): *enfriar*
cooperate (v.): *cooperar*
copious: *copioso*
copper: *cobre*
copy (v.): *copiar*
copy: *copia*
cordial: *cordial*
cordially: *cordialmente*
corduroy: *pana*
cork: *corcho*
corkscrew: *sacacorchos, tirabuzón*
corn: *maíz*
corner: *esquina*
corns: *callos*
corporation: *corporación*
corpse: *cadáver*
corpulent: *corpulento*
correct: *correcto, acertado*
correction: *corrección*
correctly: *correctamente*
correspondent: *correspondiente*
corrosive: *corrosivo*
corrupt (v.): *inficionar, malear*
corset: *corsé*
corss-eyed: *bizco*
cosmetic: *cosmético*

cost (v.): *costar*
cost: *costo, gasto*
cotton: *algodón*
cotton grower: *algodonero*
cotton swabs: *aplicadores de algodón, tapón de algodón*
cough (v.): *toser*
cough: *tos*
counselor: *consejero*
count: *conde*
countable: *contable*
counter: *mostrador*
counterbalance (v.): *contrapesar*
country: *país*
countryside: *campiña, paisaje, campo*
county: *condado*
couple (v.): *acoplar, par*
couple; two people: *pareja*
couple; a couple of: *un par de*
courage: *coraje*
course: *curso*
court (v.): *cortejar*
courteous: *cortés*
courtesy: *cortesía*
cousin: *primo-a*
cove: *cala*
cover (v.): *andar*
cover (v.): *cubrir*
covered: *cubierto*
cow: *vaca*
coward: *cobarde*
cowboy: *vaquero*
coyote: *coyote*
crab: *cangrejo*
crabs; lice: *ladillas*
crack: *agrietarse*
crack; cocaine: *crak, cocaína*
cracker: *galleta*
cradle: *cuna*
cramp; abdominal: *torsón, retortijón*
cramp; muscular: *calambre*
cramps: *calambres*
crane: *grúa*
crank: *manivela*
crash: *estrellarse*
crater: *cráter*
crawl: *arraste, arrastrarse*
crazy: *loco, alocado*
cream cheese: *queso crema*
cream: *crema*
cream; a&d: *crema de a & d*
cream; desitin: *crema de desitin*
create (v.): *crear*

creation: *creación*
creative: *creador*
creator: *creador*
creature: *criatura*
credible: *creíble*
credit card: *tarjeta de crédito*
credit: *crédito*
creed: *credo*
cretinism: *cretinismo*
crib: *cuna*
cricket: *grillo*
crime: *atentado, crimen*
criminal: *criminal*
crippled: *empedido, lisiado, cojo*
crisis: *crisis*
criterion: *criterio*
critic: *crítico*
critical: *crítico*
croak: *graznido*
crocodile: *cocodrilo*
crooked: *engañoso*
cross (v.): *cruzar*
cross out (v.): *tachar*
cross-eyed: *turnio, bizco, bisojo, ojo cruza, ojituerto*
cross: *aspa, cruzarse, cruz*
crotch: *entrepiernas*
crowd: *muchedumbre*
crown: *corona*
crucify (v.): *crucificar*
cruel: *cruel*
crumb: *migaja*
crush: *apretura*
crutches: *muletas*
cry (v.): *llorar*
cry: *grito/lloro*
cry-baby: *llorón*
crystal ball: *bola de cristal*
cuba: *cuba*
cube: *cubo*
cubic: *cúbico*
cucumber: *pepino*
culture: *cultura*
culture; blood: *cultivo de la sangre*
culture; csf: *cultivo del fluido espinal*
culture; sputum: *cultivo del esputo*
culture; throat: *cultivo de la garganta*
culture; urine: *cultivo de la orina*
cup: *taza, copa*
cupboard: *alacena*
cupful: *taza*
cura-all: *sanalotodo*
cure (v.): *curar*
cure: *cura*

curiosity: *curiosidad*
curious: *curioso*
curl: *bucle, rizo, tirabuzón*
currant: *grosella*
currency: *moneda*
current: *actual, corriente*
curse: *maldición*
curtain: *cortina, telón*
curve (v.): *encorvar*
custody: *custodia*
customs: *aduana*
customs agent: *agente de aduana, aduanero*
cut (v.): *cortar*
cut: *cortada, cortadura*
cut off (v.): *amputar*
cut oneself (v.): *cortarse*
cut out (v.): *recortar*
cute: *bonito-a*
cutlet: *chuleta*
cutting: *cortador, corte, recorte*
cyanide: *cianuro*
cyanosis: *piel azulada "blue skin", cianosis*
cycle: *ciclo*
cylinder: *cilindro*
cynical: *cínico*
cyst: *quiste*
cystitis: *cistitis*

D

dad: *papá*
daily: *cotidiano*
dairy: *lechería*
dairyman: *lechero*
daisy: *margarita*
damage: *avería*
damp: *húmedo*
dance (v.): *bailar*
dancer: *bailador, bailarina*
dandruff: *caspa*
danger: *peligro*
dangerous: *peligroso*
dare: *atreverse*
dark: *oscuro*
dart: *dardo, rehilete*
dash: *gallardía*
data: *datos*
date: *fecha*
daughter: *hija*
daughter-in-law: *nuera*
dawn: *amanecer, alba, madrugada*

day: *día*
day; after next: *pasado mañana*
day; after tomorrow: *pasado mañana*
day; any day now: *de un día para otro*
day; before last: *anteayer*
day; before yesterday: *anteayer*
day; the day after: *el día siguiente*
day; the day before: *la víspera*
days: *días*
daze (v.): *abobar*
dazed: *aturdido*
dazzle (v.): *deslumbrar*
dead: *muerto, difunto*
deaden (v.): *amortiguar*
deaden the nerve: *adormecer el nervio*
deaf: *sordo*
deafness: *sordera*
deal (v.): *tallar*
deal with: *entender en*
dean: *decano*
dear: *caro*
death: *muerte*
debate: *debate*
debilitate (v.): *debilitar*
debility: *debilidad*
debit: *débito*
debris: *despojos*
debt: *deuda*
decade: *década*
decaffeinated: *descafeinado*
decay: *decaimiento, podredumbre, carcomerse*
decayed tooth: *diente cariado*
decease: *defunción*
deceive (v.): *burlar*
december: *diciembre*
decent: *decente*
deception: *decepción*
decide (v.): *decidir*
decision: *decisión*
deck (v.): *ataviar*
declaim (v.): *declamar*
declaration: *declaración*
declare (v.): *declarar*
decline (v.): *decaer*
decorate (v.): *condecorar*
decrease: *decrecer, disminuir, mengua*
deduction: *deducción*
deep: *hondo, penetrante, profundo*
deepen (v.): *ahondar*
deer: *venado, ciervo*

defeat (v.): *derrotar*
defecate (v.): *defecar, hacer caca*
defecation: *defecación*
defect: *defecto*
defect; birth: *defecto de nacimiento*
defect; congenital: *defecto congénito*
defective: *defectuoso*
defence: *defensa*
defend (v.): *defender*
deficient: *deficiente*
deficit: *déficit*
deform (v.): *deformar*
deformed: *deforme*
deformity: *deformidad*
degeneration (v.): *degenerar*
degree: *grado*
dehydrate (v.): *dehidratar, perder fluidos del cuerpo "lose fluid from the body"*
delay: *demora*
delicious: *delicioso*
delight (v.): *deleitar*
delighted: *encantado-a*
delirious: *delirante*
delirium: *delirio*
deliver (v.): *entregar*
delivery room: *sala de alumbramientos, sala de partos, sala de aliviarse*
delivery; of a baby: *alumbramiento, el parto*
deluge: *diluvio*
demand (v.): *demandar, exigir*
demand: *demanda*
demanding: *exigente*
demented: *demente*
democracy: *democracia*
demonstrate: *demonstrativo*
den: *guarida*
density: *densidad*
dental clinic: *clinica dental*
dental: *dental*
dentist: *dentista*
denture: *dentadura, dentadura postiza*
denture; full: *dentadura completa*
denture; partial: *dentadura parcial*
deny (v.): *nebar, desautorizar*
deodorant: *desodorante*
department of social security: *departamento de seguridad social*
department: *departamento*
department; medical records: *departamento de archivo clínico*

department; medicine: *departamento de medicina*
department; mental health: *departamento de enfermedades mentales*
department; nursing: *departamento de enfermería*
department; orthopedics: *departamento de ortopedia*
department; pediatrics: *departamento de pediatría*
department; personnel: *departamento de personal*
department; social services: *departamento de servicio social*
department; surgery: *departamento de cirugía*
departure: *partida, salida*
depend; depend on (v.): *depender*
dependent: *dependiente*
deport (v.): *deportar*
deposit (v.): *depositar*
deposit: *depósito*
depressed: *deprimido*
depression: *depresión*
depth: *hondura*
dermatitis: *dermatitis*
dermatology: *dermatología*
descent: *bajada*
describe (v.): *describir*
description: *descripción*
desert (v.): *abandonar, desamparar*
desertion: *deserción*
deserve (v.): *merecer*
design: *diseño*
desire (v.): *desear, querer*
desirous: *deseoso*
desk: *escritorio*
despair: *desconsolarse*
dessert: *postre*
destination: *destino*
destroy (v.): *destruir*
detail (v.): *detallar*
detergent: *detergente*
deterioration: *deterioración, deterioramiento*
determination: *determinación*
determine (v.): *determinar*
detest (v.): *detestar*
detour: *desvío, rodeo*
detoxicate (v.): *desintoxicar*
detoxification: *desintoxicación*
develop (v.): *desarrollar*
development: *desarrollo*
deviate: *desviarse*

device: *aparato, recurso*
devil: *demonio*
devote (v.): *dedicar*
devout: *devoto*
dew: *rocío*
diabetes: *diabetes*
diabetic: *diabético*
diagnose (v.): *diagnosticar*
diagnosis: *diagnosis, diagnóstico*
diagram: *esquema*
diamond: *diamante*
diaper: *pañal*
diaper; cloth: *pañal de tela*
diaper; disposable: *pañal desechable*
diapers: *los pañales*
diaphragm: *diafragma*
diarrhea: *diarrea*
diary: *agenda*
dictionary: *diccionario*
die (v.): *morir*
diet: *dieta*
different: *diferente*
difficult: *difícil*
difficulty: *dificultad*
diffuse (v.): *difundir*
dig (v.): *cavar*
digest (v.): *digerir*
digested: *digerido*
digestible: *digestible*
digestion: *digestión*
digestive: *digestivo*
digestive system: *sistema digestivo*
digital: *digital*
dilate (v.): *dilatar*
dilation: *dilatación*
dilation of the cervix: *dilatación del cuello de la matriz*
diligent: *diligente*
dilute (v.): *diluir*
diminish (v.): *disminuir*
din: *algazara*
dine (v.): *cenar*
dining room: *comedor*
dinner: *cena, comida*
diphtheria: *difteria*
diplomat: *diplomático*
direct (v.): *dirigir, encaminar*
direct: *directo, dirigirse*
direct oneself to: *dirigirse a*
directions: *dirección, direcciones*
director: *director*
dirt: *mugre*
dirty (v.): *ensuciar*
dirty: *sucio*

disagreeable: *desagradable*
disarm (v.): *desarmar*
disaster: *desastre*
discharge (from hosp.): *dar de alta*
discharge: *descarga*
discharge: *flujo, secreciones, desechos*
discharge; ear: *desechos de los oídos*
discharge; penile: *desechos de el pene*
discharge; vaginal: *flujó vaginales, secreción vaginal (anormal)*
discipline: *disciplina*
discomfort: *molestia*
disconnect (v.): *desconectar*
discontented: *descontent-a*
discount: *descuent*
discover (v.): *descubrir*
discovery: *descubrimiento*
discretion: *discreción*
discuss (v.): *discutir*
discussion: *discusión*
disease: *enfermedad*
disease; communicable: *enfermedad transmisible*
disease; contagious: *enfermedad contagiosa*
disease; venereal: *enfermedad venérea*
disguise: *disfaz*
disgust: *disgusto*
dish (v.): *plato, manjar*
dishonor (v.): *infamar*
dishwasher: *lavaplatos*
disinfect (v.): *desinfectar*
disinfectant: *desinfectante*
disk: *disco*
dislocate (v.): *dislocar, descoyuntar*
disobey (v.): *desobedecer*
disposable diapers: *los pañales desechables*
disposable: *disponible*
dissolve (v.): *disolver*
distance: *distancia, lejanía, trecho*
distant: *distante*
distinguish (v.): *distinguir*
distribute (v.): *distribuir*
distribution: *distribución*
disturb (v.): *desasosegar*
ditch: *foso*
divan: *diván*
dive: *bucear, zambullirse*
diverticulitis: *diverticulitis*
divide (v.): *dividir, compartir*
divine: *divino*
division: *división*

divorced: *divorciado*
dizziness: *mareo, vértigo*
dizzy: *mareado*
do (v.): *hacer*
do you have…: *¿tiene usted…?*
docile: *dócil*
doctor; M.D.: *médico*
doctor; Ph.D. or M.D.: *doctor*
document: *documento*
dog: *perro*
doll: *muñeca*
dollar: *dólar*
dolphin: *delfín*
donation: *dádiva*
donkey: *anso, borrico, burro*
door: *puerta*
dormitory: *dormitorio*
dose: *dosis, toma*
double: *doble*
double room: *cuarto doble*
doubt (v.): *dudar*
doubt: *duda*
doubtful: *dudoso*
douche: *ducha, lavado vaginal*
dough: *masa*
dove: *paloma*
down: *abajo*
down's syndrome: *minos mongolicos*
downstairs: *escalera abajo*
doze (v.): *dormitar*
dozen: *docena*
drag (v.): *arrastrar*
drain: *albañal*
drain cleaner: *límpiador de tuberia, destapador de cañería*
drama: *drama*
dramamine: *dramamina*
dramatization: *dramatismo*
draw (v.): *dibujar*
draw up (v.): *redactar*
drawer: *cajón*
drawing: *dibujo*
dread: *pavor*
dream (v.): *soñar*
dream: *ensueño*
dress (a person) (v.): *vestir*
dress up: *aderezarse*
dress: *vestido, atuendo, vestirse*
dressing room: *cuarto de vestir, vestidor, vestuario*
dressing: *vendaje*
dressmaker: *costurer*
drift: *derivarse*
drill (v.): *taladrar*

drill: *taladro*
drink (v.): *beber*
drink; alcoholic: *bebida alcohólica*
drip (v.): *gotear*
drip: *escurrirse, gotearse*
drive (v.): *manejar*
drive mad (v.): *enloquecer*
driver: *conductor, muletero (horses), cochero (coach)*
driver's license: *licencia de manejar*
driver; of car: *chofer, cochero*
drive-in theater: *auto-teatro, motocine*
driving: *manedando*
drizzle: *llovizna*
drool (v.): *babear*
drool: *baba*
dropper: *gotero*
drops: *gotas*
drown (v.): *ahogar*
drowsy: *soñoliento, modorro*
drug (v.): *narcotizar*
drug addict: *drogadicto*
drug addiction: *dependencia famacológica, drogadicción*
drug: *droga*
druggist: *boticario, droguista*
drugstore: *botica, farmacia*
drum: *tambor*
drunk: *borracho, bolo, beodo*
drunkard: *espita*
dry (v.): *secar*
dry: *seco, seca, enjuto*
dry up: *desecarse, marchitar, resecarse*
dual: *doble*
duck (v.): *chapuzar*
duck: *pato, ánade*
duel: *duelo*
dull: *deslucido*
dumb: *mudo*
dung: *bosta*
durability: *durabilidad*
durable: *durable*
duration: *duración*
during: *durante, mientras*
dust: *espolvorear, polvo*
duty: *deber*
dwarf (v.): *empequeñecer*
dwarf: *enano*
dye (v.): *teñir*
dying: *agonizante*
dysentery: *disentería*
dyslexia: *dislexia*

E

e.c.g.; electrocardiogram: *electrocardiógrafo*
e.k.g.; electrocardiogram: *electrocardiógrafo*
each: *cada*
eager: *anhelante*
eagerness: *anhelo*
eagle: *águila*
ear; inner: *oído, sentido*
ear; outer: *oreja*
earache: *dolor del oído, otitis*
earlier: *más temprano*
early: *temprano*
earn (v.): *granjear*
earnest: *sincero-a*
earnings: *ganacias*
earring: *arete*
earth: *tierra*
earwax (cerumen): *cera, cerilla*
ease: *desenvoltura,facilidad*
easily: *fácilmente*
east: *este, oriente*
easy: *fácil*
eat (v.): *comer*
eatable: *comestible*
eaves: *alero*
ecg; electrocardiogram: *electrocardiógrafo*
echo (v.): *retumbar*
echo: *eco*
ecology: *ecologia*
economy: *ahorro, economía*
ectopic: *ectópico*
eczema: *eczema*
edema: *hinchazón de las piernas "swelling of legs"*
edge: *borde*
edges: *confínes*
educable: *educable*
education: *educación*
eel: *anguila*
effect: *efecto*
efficient: *eficaz, eficiente*
effort: *esfuerzo*
egg: *huevo*
egg; fried: *huevo frito*
egg; hard-boiled: *huevo duro*
egg; scrambled: *huevo revuelto*
egg; soft-boiled: *huevo pasado por agua*

egg; yolk: *yema del huevo*
egotism: *egoismo*
eight: *ocho*
eighteen: *dieci-ocho*
eighth: *octavo*
eighty: *ochenta*
either: *tampoco*
ejaculation: *eyaculación*
eject (v.): *desalojar*
ekg; electrocardiogram:
 electrocardiógrafo
elbow: *codo*
elderly: *anciano, viejo*
electric shaver: *máquina de afeitar*
electrician: *electricista*
elegant: *elegante*
elephantiasis: *elefantiasis*
elevation: *elevación*
elevator: *ascensor, elevador*
eleven: *once*
eliminate (v.): *eliminar*
elimination: *eliminación*
elsewhere: *en otra parte*
embolism: *embolismo*
emergency: *emergencia*
emergency room: *sala de emergencia*
emesis basin: *tazón para vómitar*
emetic: *emético*
emotion: *emoción*
emotional: *emocionable, emocional*
empathy: *empatía, enfasis*
emphysema: *enfisema*
employee: *empleado-a*
employment: *empleo, trabajo empty vacío*
empty (v.): *vaciar*
empty: *vacío-a*
enamel: *esmalte*
encephalitis: *encefalitis*
encephalomyelitis: *encefalomielitis*
end (v.): *terminar*
end: *fin*
endangered: *en peligro*
endocarditis: *endocarditis*
endocrine: *endocrina*
endocrinology: *endocrinología*
endure (v.): *durar*
enema: *enema, lavado, lavativa*
enemy: *enemigo*
engineer: *ingeniero*
engineering: *ingeniería*
english: *inglés*
enjoy oneself (v.): *divertirse*
enough: *bastante, suficiente*

enriched: *enriquecido*
enter (v.): *entrar, pasar*
enteritis: *enteritis*
entrance: *entrada*
entry: *zaguán*
envelope: *sobre*
envious: *envidioso*
environment: *ambiente*
ephedrine: *efedrina*
epidemic: *epidémico*
epilepsy: *epilepsia*
episiotomy: *episiotomia*
episode: *episodio*
equal: *igual, par*
equipment: *equipo*
erase (v.): *borrar*
err: *descarriarse*
eruption: *erupción*
escape (v.): *escapar*
escapee: *escapado, evadido*
escort: *escolta*
eskimo: *esquimal*
esophagus: *esófago*
especially: *especialmente, sobre todo,
 máxime*
essential: *esencial*
establishment: *establecimiento*
eternity: *eternidad*
eustacion tube: *tubo de eustaquio*
evacuate (v.): *evacuar*
evacuation: *evacuación*
evaluate (v.): *evaluar*
evaluation: *evaluación*
evasion: *evasión*
even: *igual*
evening: *tarde*
every: *cada, todo*
everywhere: *por todas partes*
evolution: *evolución*
exactly: *exactamente*
examination: *examen*
examine (v.): *examinar*
example: *ejemplo*
excellence: *excelencia*
excellent: *excelente*
except: *excepto*
except for: *con excepción de*
exception: *excepción*
excess: *exceso*
excited: *gitado*
excrement: *excremento*
exercise (v.): *ejercer, hacer los
 ejercicios*
exercise: *ejercicio, exercicio*

exhale (v.): *exhalar*
exist (v.): *existir*
existence: *existencia*
exit: *salida*
expectation: *expectación*
expectoration: *expectoración*
expense: *gasto*
expensive: *caro, cara*
experience (v.): *experimentar*
experience: *experiencia*
explanation: *explicación*
explication: *explicación*
exploration: *exploración*
exploratory: *exploratorio*
explore (v.): *explorar*
explosion: *explosión*
express (v.): *expresar*
extra: *extra*
extract (v.): *extraer*
extraction: *extracción*
extrauterine: *extrauterino*
extremity: *extremidad*
eye exam: *examen de los ojos*
eye: *ojo*
eye socket: *cuenca de los ojos*
eyeball: *globo del ojo*
eyebrow: *ceja*
eyeglasses: *anteojos, espejuelos, gafas*
eyelash: *pestaña*
eyelid: *párpado*
eyes: *ojos*
eyetooth: *colmillo*

F

fable: *fábula*
fabric: *tela*
face (v.): *enfrentar*
face down (on one's stomach): *boca abajo*
face: *rostro, cara*
face up (on one's back): *boca arriba*
facilitate (v.): *facilitar*
facility: *facilidad*
facing: *cara a*
fact: *dato*
factor: *factor*
factory: *fábrica*
faculty: *facultad*
fade (v.): *desteñir*
fail (v.): *fracasar*
failure: *fracaso, malogro*

faint (v.): *desmayar, desfallecer*
fainting spell: *desmayarse, desmayo*
fair: *bonancible*
fairy: *hada*
faith: *fe*
fall (autumn): *ontoño*
fall (v.): *caer*
fall asleep (v.): *dormir*
fall asleep: *adormecerse*
fall down: *caerse*
fall guy: *cabeza de turco*
fall in love: *enamorarse*
fall; season: *otoñal*
fall; water: *caída, caída de agua*
fallible: *falible*
fallopian tube: *tubo falopio, tramp de falopio*
false: *falso*
false teeth: *dentadura postiza*
false; imitation: *postiza*
fame: *celebridad*
familiar: *familiar*
familiarity: *familiaridad*
family: *familia*
famous: *famoso-a*
fan: *abanico, ventilador*
far away: *lejos*
far: *lejos*
farce: *cachondeo*
farewell: *despedida*
farm: *granja*
farmer: *hacendado, agricultor*
fart (slang): *pedo, gas*
fashion: *moda*
fast forward: *avance rápido*
fast: *rápido*
fast-food restaurant: *rotisería*
fasting: *ayuno*
fat (adjective): *gordo, gordura,*
fat (noun): *manteca, grasa*
fat free: *sin grasa "without grease"*
fat; to get fat (v.): *engordar*
fatalism: *fatalismo*
fate: *azar, fatalidad, sino*
father: *padre, papá*
father-in-law: *suegro*
fatigue: *fatiga*
fatten (v.): *cebar*
faucet: *grifo*
fault: *culpa, falla, falta*
favor: *favor*
favorite: *favorito*
favoritism: *favoritismo*
fear: *miedo*

february: *febrero*
fecundation: *fecundación*
federation: *federación*
fee: *cuenta*
feed (v.): *alimentar, dar de comer*
feed oneself: *alimentarse*
feel; emotion (v.): *sentir*
feel; touch (v.): *tocar*
feeling: *sentimiento*
feet: *pies*
female: *hembra*
femininity: *feminidad*
fence in (v.): *cercar*
fertile: *fecundo, fértil*
fester: *enconarse*
fetus: *feto*
feudalism: *feudalismo*
fevers: *fiebre, calentura*
few; a few; some: *unas, una(-as), pocos(-as)*
fiancé: *novio*
fiancée: *novia*
fibrillation: *fibrilación*
fibroma: *fibroma*
fibrous: *fibroso*
fifteen: *quince*
fifty: *cincuenta*
fig: *higo*
fight (v.): *batallar*
file (v.): *archivar*
fill (a tooth) (v.): *empastar*
fill (v.): *llenar*
fillet: *filete*
filling (of teeth): *empaste, lleno*
film: *filmar, pelicula*
filth: *inmundicia, porquería*
fin: *aleta*
finally: *finalmente, por fin*
find (v.): *encontrar, hallar*
find out (v.): *averiguar*
fine art: *bellas artes*
fine: *fino*
finger: *dedo*
finger; index: *dedo índice*
finger; little: *dedo meñique*
finger; middle: *dedo medio*
finger; ring: *dedo anular*
fingernail: *uña*
finish (v.): *acabar, terminar*
finished: *terminado-a*
finishing, ending: *terminand*
fire: *fuego*
fireman: *bombero*
firm; business: *casa comercial, empresa, entidad*
firm; not soft: *duro*
firmament: *firmamento*
first floor: *plantabaja*
first name: *nombre*
first: *primer, primero*
fish: *pescado*
fisherman: *pescador*
fissure: *quebradura*
fist: *puño*
fistula: *fístula*
fit (v.): *caber*
five: *cinco*
fix (v.): *arreglar*
flag: *bandera*
flame: *llama*
flank pain: *dolor de flanco, dolor de lado*
flash (v.): *relampaguear*
flat: *bemol*
flat foot: *pie plano*
flatter (v.): *adular, halagar, lisonjear*
flattered: *complacido-a*
flatulate (pass gas) (v.): *echar aire, tirarse flato*
flatulence: *flatulencia*
flavour: *sabor*
flee: *fugarse*
flesh: *carne*
flexibility: *flexibilidad*
flexible: *flexible*
flexion: *flexión*
flight: *fuga*
float (v.): *flotar*
float: *corcho*
flood: *arriarse*
floor: *piso*
flour: *harina*
flour; corn: *harina de maíz*
flour; wheat: *harina de trigo*
flow (v.): *afluir*
flower: *flor*
flowers: *flores*
flu: *gripe, influenza*
fluff: *borra*
fluid: *fluido*
flushing (blushing): *bochornos*
flute: *flauta, gaita*
flutter (v.): *aletear*
fly (v.): *volar*
fly; insect: *mosca*
foam: *espuma*
fog: *niebla*
fold: *arruga*

follow a diet: *seguir una dieta*
follow: *seguir, seguirse*
fomentation: *fomento*
fontanel: *mollera, fontanela*
food: *alimento, comida*
fool: *mentecato*
foolishness: *tontería*
foot: *pie*
football: *fútbol*
footstep: *pisada*
for a long time: *por mucho tiempo*
for: *para, por*
for, in order to: *para*
force: *fuerza*
forceful: *enérgico*
forceps: *forceps*
foreign body: *cuerpo extranjero*
forearm: *antebrazo*
forecast: *previsión*
forehead: *frente*
forest: *bosque, monte alto, selva*
forget (v.): *olvidar de*
fork: *tenedor, bifurcación*
form (v.): *formar*
form: *forma, formulario*
formal dinner: *banquete*
formality: *formalidad*
formation: *formación*
formula: *fórmula*
fortunately: *afortunadamente*
fortune: *dineral, fortuna*
forty: *cuarenta*
forward: *encabeza, adelante*
founder: *poblador*
fountain: *fuente*
four: *cuatro*
fourteen: *catorce*
fowl: *ave*
fracture (v.): *fracturar*
fracture: *quebradura, fractura, rotura de hueso*
fragile: *frágil*
fragility: *fragilidad*
fragment: *fragmento*
frame: *bastidor*
france: *francia*
fraud: *farsante*
freckles: *pecas*
free; no cost: *gratis*
freeze (v.): *congelar*
frequency: *frecuencia*
frequent: *frecuente*
frequently: *con frecuencia, frecuentemente*

fresh: *fresco*
friction: *fricción*
friday: *viernes*
fried: *frito*
fried potato: *papa frita*
friend: *amigo-a*
friendly: *amigable*
frighten (v.): *asustar*
frightened: *asustado*
frog: *rana*
frolic (v.): *retozar*
from: *desde, de*
front: *delantero*
frost: *escarcha*
frown: *ceño*
frozen: *congelado, congelada, helado*
frugal: *parco*
fruit: *fruta*
fry: *freír*
fuel: *combustible*
full denture: *dentadura completa*
full: *harto*
function (v.): *funcionar*
function: *funcionamiento, función*
functionary: *funcionario*
funds: *fondos*
funeral: *fúnebre*
funerary: *funerario*
fungi: *hongos*
funnel: *embudo*
funny: *bufón, chusco, gracioso, chistoso*
fur: *pelaje*
furious: *furioso*
furnace: *horno*
furnished: *amueblado*
furniture: *mobiliar, mueble*
fuss: *aspaviento*
fussy: *fastidioso*
future: *futuro, porvenir*

G

gag: *mordaza*
gain: *ganacia*
gain weight (v.): *aumentar de peso*
gait: *andadura*
gall bladder attack: *ataque de la vesícular biliar*
gall bladder: *vesícula biliar, hiel*
gall stone: *cálculo biliar, piedra biliar, piedras de la hiel*
gallant: *galante*

gallon: *galón*
gamma globulin: *gamaglobulina, globulina gamma*
gang: *banda*
gangrene: *gangrena*
gap: *boquete*
garage: *cochera, garaje*
garden: *jardín*
gardener: *jardinero*
gargle (v.): *hacer gárgaras*
gargling: *gárgara*
garlic: *ajo*
gas: *gas*
gash: *cuchillada*
gasoline: *gasolina*
gasp (v.): *boquear*
gastritis: *gastritis*
gastroenterology: *gastroenterología*
gastrointestinal: *gastrointestinal*
gastroscopy: *gastroscopia*
gather (v.): *agregar*
gauge (v.): *calibrar*
gauze: *gasa*
gauze: *gasa*
gay; festive: *alegre, festivo*
gay; homosexual: *homosexual*
gee!: *¡arre!*
gelatin: *gelatina*
generality: *generalidad*
generally: *generalmente*
generosity: *generosidad*
generous: *generoso*
genetic: *genético*
genious: *genio*
genital organs: *órganos genitales*
gentility: *gentilidad*
gentleman; mr.; sir: *señor, sr.*
genuine: *genuino*
geography: *geografia*
geography: *geografía*
geriatrics: *geriatría*
germ: *germen*
german: *alemán*
german measles: *sarampion aleman, rubéola*
gestation: *gestación*
gesture: *ademán*
get (v.): *conseguir*
get alarmed: *sorprenderse, azorarse*
get angry: *airarse, encolerizarse, enojarse*
get annoyed: *fastidiarse*
get better (v.): *mejorar*
get dressed (v.): *vestirse*

get excited: *agitarse*
get on (v.): *congeniar*
get tired: *cansarse*
get up (v.): *levantarse*
get used: *habituarse*
get wet: *mojarse*
ghost: *fantasma, espectro*
gibe: *burla*
gift: *regalo, don*
gift shop: *tienda de regalos*
gifted: *dotado*
gifts: *regalos, dotes*
gin: *ginebra, desmotadera de algodón*
ginger: *jengibre*
gingivitis: *gingivitis*
giraffe: *jirafa*
girl: *muchacha*
girlfriend: *novia*
give (v.): *dar*
give an injection: *poner una inyección*
give birth (v.): *dar a luz "give to the light"*
give way: *franquearse*
gladly: *con gusto*
glance: *ojeada*
gland: *glándula*
glass: *vidrio, cristal*
glass; drinking: *vaso, copa, copita*
glass; of water: *vaso de agua*
glaucoma: *glaucoma*
gloomy: *mohino*
glorious: *glorioso*
glory: *gloria*
glove: *guante*
gloves: *guantes*
glue (v.): *pegar*
glutton: *gloton*
glycerin: *glicerina*
go (v.): *ir(se), andar*
go around (v.): *orillar*
go away: *andarse, ausentarse*
go down (v.): *bajar*
go on (v.): *ir sobre*
go out (v.): *salir*
go through: *revolver en*
go to bed (v.): *acostarse*
goal: *gol, meta*
god: *dios*
godchild: *ahijado-a*
goddaughter: *ahijada*
godfather: *padrino*
godly: *pío, devoto*
godmother: *madrina*

godsend: *cosa llovida del cielo, bendición*
godson: *ahijado*
going: *ida*
goiter: *bocio, papera*
gold: *dorado, oro*
golf: *golf*
gong: *canción, batintín*
gonorrhea: *gonorrea*
good: *bien, bueno, buena*
good time: *juerga*
goodbye: *adiós*
goodness: *bondad*
goofy: *tonto (slang), mentecato*
gopher: *ardilla de tierra*
gorilla: *gorila*
gossip (v.): *comadrear*
gout: *gota*
govern (v.): *regir*
gown: *camisón, manto*
grab (v.): *agarrar de*
grab bar: *barra de agarrarse*
grace: *garbo, gracia*
gractous: *gracioso*
gradual: *gradual*
grain: *granos*
gram: *gramo*
gramar: *gramática*
granddaughter: *nieta*
grandfather: *abuelo*
grandma: *abuelita*
grandmother: *abuela*
grandson: *nieto*
granny: *abuelita*
grant: *beca*
grape: *uva*
grapefruit juice: *jugo de toronja*
grapefruit: *toronja, pomelo*
grass: *pasto, césped, hierba*
grassy: *con hierba*
grate (v.): *rallar*
grave: *fosa, sepultura*
gravity: *gravedad*
gray: *gris*
grayhound: *galgo*
graze (v.): *pacer*
grease (v.): *engrasar*
grease: *grasa*
greasy: *grasoso, grasient*
greece: *grecia*
greed: *codicia*
green been: *habichuela verde*
green peas: *arvejas*
green: *verde, verduras, bisoño*

greet (v.): *saludar*
greeting: *saludo*
gregarious: *gregario*
grey: *gris, rucio*
grey hair: *canas*
grey-headed: *cano*
grief: *desgarro*
grieve (v.): *apenar*
grill: *parrilla*
grin: *rictus*
grind (v.): *moler*
grocer: *abacero*
groceries: *abarrotes*
groin: *empeine*
groin: *ingle*
groove (v.): *acanalar*
ground floor: *planta baja*
group: *agrupación*
grove: *arboleda*
grow (v.): *crecer*
grow thin: *chuparse*
growl (v.): *gruñir*
growth: *crecimiento*
grub: *gorgojo*
grumble (v.): *rezongar*
grunt (v.): *refunfuñar*
guarantee: *guarantor*
guard: *guarda*
guardian: *custodio*
guess (v.): *barruntar, conjeturar, creer*
guess: *conjetura*
guest: *convidado, invitado*
guide (v.): *gobernar*
guide: *guía*
guideline: *pauta*
guilt: *culpabilidad*
guilty: *culpable*
guitar: *guitarra*
gulf: *golfo*
gulp: *sorbo, trago*
gum (v.): *engomar*
gum: *encía, goma de pegar, chicle*
gums: *encías*
gums; infection: *infeccion de las encias*
gums; inflamed: *encias inflamadas*
gun: *escopeta, fusil, revólver, pistola*
gun shot: *escopetazo, tiro de fusil*
gunboat: *coñonero*
gunshot wound: *escopetazo*
gush (v.): *chorrear*
gynecology: *ginecología*

H

habit: *hábito*
hail (v.): *granizar*
hair loss: *pérdida del pelo*
hair: *pelo, cabello*
hairbrush: *cepillo para el cabello*
hairless: *calvo*
haiti: *haití*
half: *medio, mitad*
halitosis: *halitosis, mal aliento*
hall: *vestíbulo*
hallucinate (v.): *alucinar*
halluctnation: *alucinación*
hallway: *pasillo, zaguán*
halo: *aureola*
halt: *apeadero*
halter: *cabestro*
ham: *jamón*
hamburger: *hamburguesa*
hamlet: *caserío*
hammer (v.): *martillar*
hamper: *cesto*
hand (noun): *mano*
hand (v.): *entregar*
hand over (v.): *ceder*
handbook: *manual*
handcuff (v.): *esposar*
handful: *manojo*
handicap: *impedimento*
handkerchief: *pañuelo*
handle: *agarradero, asa*
handrail: *pasamano*
handsome: *guapo, garrido*
hang (v.): *ahorcar*
hanger: *colgadero*
hanging: *colgante*
happen (v.): *pasar, suceder, acaecer*
happiness: *alegría, bienandanza, felicidad*
happy: *alegre*
harass (v.): *afanar*
hard: *duro, dura, empedernido, endurecido*
hare: *liebre*
harm (v.): *damnificar, lacrar*
harm: *daño, deterimento*
harm oneself (v.): *hacerse daño, dañarse*
harmonious: *armonioso*
harness: *arneses*
harpoon: *arpón*
harvest (v.): *cosecha, cosechar*

harvester: *cosechero*
hastily: *apurado, apurada*
hasty: *precipitado*
hat: *sombrero*
hate (v.): *aborrecer*
hateful: *aborrecible*
hatmaker: *sombrerero*
have a cold (v.): *tener catarro, tener un resfriado*
have breakfast (v.): *tomar el desayuno, desayunar*
have fun (v.): *divertirse*
have good vision (v.): *tener buena vista*
have lunch (v.): *almorzar*
have pain (v.): *tener dolor*
have to: *haber de*
have worth (v.): *valer*
have you; do you have…: *¿tiene usted…?*
have you… (possession): *tiene*
have; possess (v.): *tener, haber*
hay fever: *fiebre de heno*
hay: *heno*
he: *él*
head (v.): *encabecar*
head: *cabeza*
head of bed: *cabecera*
headache: *dolor de cabeza, jaqueca*
headline: *cabecera*
health: *salud*
healthy: *sano, salubre, saludable*
hear (v.): *oír*
hearing aid: *aparato para la sordera, audiófono*
hearing: *oída, audición*
hearing test: *examen de audición*
heart ache: *angustia, dolor del corazón*
heart attack: *ataque al corazón*
heart broken: *muerto de pena, corazón roto*
heart burn: *acedía, agruras*
heart: *corazón*
heart disease: *enfermedad del corazón*
heart failure: *falla cardiaca, falla del corazón*
heart murmur: *soplo del corazón*
heat (v.): *acalorar*
heat: *calor*
heating pad: *almohadilla eléctrica*
heaviness: *pesadez*
heavy: *pesado-a, grave*
heel: *talón, taco, tacón*

height: *altura*
hell: *infierno*
hello: *¡hola!*
help (v.): *ayudar*
help: *ayuda*
hematchezia (stool with blood): *desposiones con sangre*
hematology: *hematologia*
hemetemesis (vomit with blood): *vómito con sangre*
hemophilia: *hemofilia*
hemoptesis (cough up blood): *tose sangre*
hemorrhage: *hemorragia*
hemorrhoids: *almorranas, hemorroides*
hepatitis: *hepatitis*
her: *ella*
herb: *yerba*
here: *aquí, acá*
hereditaty: *hereditario*
hernia: *hernia*
heroin: *heroína*
heroine: *heroína*
herpe; genital: *herpes genital*
herpes: *herpes*
herring: *arenque*
hiccups: *hipo*
hidden: *oculto*
hide (v.): *desaparecer*
high: *alto*
high blood pressure: *alta presión, presion alta*
high blood sugar: *alta azúcar en la sangre*
high chair: *silla alta*
high road: *camino real*
high school: *escuela de segunda enseñanza*
high society: *alta sociedad, gan mundo*
hill: *cerro*
him: *él, le*
hinge: *bisagra*
hip: *cadera*
hippopotamus: *hipopótamo*
his: *su de el*
hispanic: *hispano*
hiss (v.): *chiflar*
history: *historia*
hit: *golpe*
hit; punch (v.): *golpear, pegar*
hives; urticaria: *urticaria, ronchas*
hoard (v.): *atesorar*

hoarse: *afónico*
hoarseness: *ronquera*
hobble: *manea*
hobby: *distracción*
hockey: *hockey*
hoist: *cabria*
hold (v.): *desempeñar*
hold onto (v.): *agarrar de*
holdup: *atraco*
hole: *agujero, hoyo, piquera*
holiday: *fiesta, asueto*
holland: *holanda*
hollow: *cuenca*
homage: *homenaje*
home (v.): *hogar*
home: *casa*
home; domicile: *domicillo*
homemaker: *ama de casa*
homeopath: *homeópata*
honest: *honesto, honesta*
honey: *miel*
honor: *honor*
hood: *caperuza*
hook: *anzuelo*
hop: *brinco*
hope (v.): *esperar*
hope: *esperanza*
hopeless: *sin esperanza*
horizon: *horizonte*
horn: *claxon*
horny: *calloso*
horror: *horror*
horse: *caballo*
hospital: *hospital*
hospitality: *hospitalidad*
hospitalization: *hospitalización*
hospitalize (v.): *hospitalizar*
hospitatization insurance: *seguro de hospitalización*
host: *anfitrión*
hostage: *rehén*
hot: *caliente*
hot flashes: *los calores, las llamaradas*
hot pack: *emplasto caliente*
hot water bottle (bag): *bolsa de agua caliente*
hotel: *hotel, parador*
hound (v.): *acosar*
hour: *hora*
house: *casa, quinta, sala*
housewife: *ama de casa*
hover: *cernirse*
how: *¿cómo?*
how far?: *¿hasta dónde?*

how long?: *¿cuánto tiempo?*
how many times?: *¿cuántas veces?*
how many?: *¿cuántos?*
how much is...?: *¿a cómo es...?*
how much?: *¿cuánto?*
how often do you... ?: *¿qué tan seguido...?*
how old?: *¿cuántas años?*
how's everything?: *¿qué tal?*
however: *sin embargo*
hug: *abrazo*
hum (v.): *tararear*
human: *humano*
humanism: *humanismo*
humanity: *humanidad*
humble: *abismar, terrero*
humidifier: *humidificador*
humidity: *humedad*
humor: *humorismo*
humorousness: *humorismo*
hump: *joroba*
hunchback: *corcovado*
hundrend; one: *cien*
hungary: *hungría*
hunger: *hambre*
hungry: *hambrienta*
hunt (v.): *cazar*
hunter: *cazador*
hurry: *apresuramiento*
hurt: *duele*
hurt oneself (v.): *dañarse, hacerse daño*
husband: *esposo, marido*
hut: *barraca*
hydrophobia: *hidrofobia, rabia*
hydrotherapy: *hidroterapia*
hygiene: *higiene*
hymn: *himno*
hyperactive: *hiperactivo*
hypertension: *altatension, hipertensión*
hyperventilation: *altaperventilación, hiperventilación*
hypnosis: *hipnosis*
hypochondria: *hipocondria*
hypochondriac: *hipocondriáco*
hypochondriasis: *hipocondriasis*
hypodermic: *hipodérmica*
hypotension: *hipotensión*
hypothesis: *hipótesis*
hypoventilation: *hipoventilación, hipoventilización*
hysterectomy: *histerectomía*
hysteria: *histeria*

I

I (person): *yo*
I have...: *yo tengo...*
I want...: *yo quiero...*
I need...: *yo necisito...*
I.U.D.: *aparato intrauterino, dispositivo intrauterino (D.I.U.)*
I.V. fluids: *suero intravenoso*
I.O.U.: *pagaré*
iraq: *irak*
iran: *irán*
ice cream: *helado*
ice: *hielo*
iceland: *islandia*
idea: *idea*
ideal: *ideal*
identification: *identificación*
identity: *identidad*
idiosyncrasy: *idiosincracia*
idiot: *lelo*
idle: *bribón*
idleness: *ociosidad*
if (whether): *si*
if: *cuando*
if not: *cuando no*
ignoble: *innoble*
ignorance: *ignorancia*
ignorant: *ignorante*
ignore (v.): *desconocer, ignorar*
ill: *enfermo*
illegal: *desaguisado, ilegal*
illness: *enfermedad*
illuminate (v.): *lucir, iluminar*
illusion: *ilusión*
illusionism: *ilusionismo*
image: *estampa, imagen*
imagination: *imaginación*
imagine (v.): *imaginar*
imagine: *figurarse, imaginarse, representarse*
imitate (v.): *imitar, remedar*
immediate: *inmediato*
immense: *inmenso*
immersion: *inmersión*
immigration: *inmigración*
imminence: *inminencia*
imminent: *inminente*
immobility: *inmovilidad*
immoble: *inmóvil, inmovible*
immortal: *inmortal*
immunity: *inmunidad*

immunization: *immunización*
immunize (v.): *inmunizar*
immunology: *inmunología*
impact: *impacto, choque*
impacted: *impactado*
impacted tooth: *muela impactado*
impacted wisdom tooth: *muela del juicio impactado*
impassable: *impasible*
impatient: *impaciente*
impediment: *impedimento*
impel (v.): *impulsar*
imperfect: *imperfeco*
impertinent: *impertinente*
impetigo: *impétigo*
impetuous: *impetuoso*
implement: *implemento*
implore (v.): *implorar*
import (v.): *importar*
importance: *importancia*
important: *importancia, importante*
impose (v.): *imponer*
imposed: *impuesto*
imposition: *abuso*
impossibility: *imposibilidad*
impossible: *imposible*
impotence: *impotencia*
impregnate (v.): *embarazar*
imprint (v.): *imprimir*
improbability: *improbabilidad*
improbable: *improbable*
improper: *impropio*
improve (v.): *mejorar*
imprudence: *imprudencia*
imprudent: *procaz*
impulse: *impulso*
impure: *impuro*
in a hurry: *apurado-a*
in: *a, en, dentro, dentro de*
in addition...: *además*
in any case: *en todo caso*
in front : *delante*
in front of: *enfrente de*
in order: *para que, por*
in reality: *en realidad*
in spite: *a pesar de*
in this manner: *de esta manera*
in tune: *entonado*
in vain: *en vano*
inaccessible: *inaccesible*
inaction: *inacción*
inaugurate (v.): *inaugurar*
incapable: *incapaz*
incapacity: *incapacidad*

incense: *incienso*
inch: *pulgada*
incision: *incisión*
incisive: *incisivo*
incisor: *incisivo*
incite (v.): *azuzar*
inclination: *inclinación*
incline (v.): *inclinar*
include (v.): *incluir*
included: *incluso*
incoherent: *incoherente*
incommunicable: *incomunicable*
incomparable: *incomparable*
incompetent: *incompetente*
incomplete: *imcompleto*
incomprehensible: *incomprensible*
incontinence: *incontinencia*
inconvenience: *desacomodo*
incorrect: *incorrecto*
incorrigible: *incorregible*
increase; augment (v.): *aumenter, acrecentar*
incredible: *increíble*
incubation: *incubación*
incubator: *incubadora*
incurable: *incurable*
indecision: *indecisión*
indefinite: *indeterminado*
independence: *independencia*
independent: *independiente*
index: *indice*
indian: *indio*
indicatable: *indicable*
indicate (v.): *denotar, indicar*
indication: *indicación*
indicator: *indicador*
indifference: *indiferencia, desamor "do not love"*
indifferent: *indiferente, estoico*
indigence: *indigencia*
indigenous; native: *autóctono, indígena*
indigestible: *indigestible*
indigestion: *indigestión*
indirect: *indirecto, indirecta*
indiscreet: *descosido, indiscreto, parlanchín*
indispensible: *imprescindible, indispensable*
indisposition: *indisposición*
indistinct: *indistinto*
individual: *individual*
indomitable: *indomable*
indulgence: *indulgencia*

industrious: *industrioso*
industry: *industria*
inefficient: *ineficiente*
inept: *inepto*
inexcusable: *imperdonable*
infallible: *infalible*
infamous: *infame*
infamy: *infamia*
infancy: *infancia, pañales*
infant: *criatura, nene, nena, infante*
infect (v.): *infectar*
infection: *infección*
infectious mononucleosis: *mono-nucleosis infecciosa*
inferior: *inferior, desaventajado*
infidelity: *infidelidad*
infinite: *infinito*
infinity: *infinidad*
infirmary: *enfermería*
infirmity: *enfermedad*
inflamed: *inflamado*
inflammation: *inflamación*
inflexible: *inflexible*
influence (v.): *incidir*
influential: *influyente*
influenza: *influenza*
inform (v.): *cerciorar, enterar, informar*
information: *información*
informed: *informado-a*
informer: *delator, informador*
infraction: *infracción*
infuse (v.): *infundir*
ingenious: *ingenioso, ingenuo*
ingeuousness: *ingenuidad*
ingredient: *ingrediente*
ingrown nail: *uñero*
ingrown toenail: *uña enterrada, uña encarnada*
inguinal: *ingle, la región inguinal*
inhalation: *inhalación*
inhale; inspire (v.): *aspirar, inhalar*
inherent: *inherente*
inheritance: *patrimonio*
inhibit (v.): *inhibir*
inhuman: *inhumano*
initial: *inicial*
inject (v.): *inyectar*
injection: *inyección*
injection; booster: *inyección secundaria*
injection; im: *inyección intramuscular*
injection; iv: *inyección intravenosa*

injection; sq: *inyección subcutánea*
injure (v.): *dañar, lastimar*
injury: *daño, herida, lesión*
ink: *tinta*
inn: *fonda*
innocence: *inocencia*
innovation: *innovación*
inoculate (v.): *inocular*
inoculation: *inoculación*
inoperable: *inoperable*
inquire (v.): *inguirir*
inquiry: *encuesta, pesquisa*
insane: *loco*
insanity: *locura*
inscription: *inscripción*
insect: *insecto*
insensibility: *insensibilidad*
insensible: *insensible*
inseparable: *inseparable*
insert (v.): *insertar, meter*
inside: *adentro, dentro*
inside of: *dentro de*
insidiuous: *insidioso*
insignificant: *insignificante*
insinuate (v.): *insinuar*
insipid: *desabrido, insipido*
insipidity: *insulsez*
insist (v.): *insistir*
insistence: *insistencia*
insole: *plantilla*
insolent: *insolente*
insomnia: *insomnio*
inspect (v.): *inspeccionar*
inspection: *inspección*
inspiration: *inspiración, numen*
inspire (v.): *insprirar*
inspired: *genial*
inspite of: *apesarde*
instability: *inestabilidad*
install (v.): *instalar*
installation: *instalación*
instance: *instancia*
instant: *instante*
instead: *envez de, en lugar de*
instep: *empeine*
instinct: *instinto*
institution: *institución*
instruct (v.): *aleccionar*
instruction: *instrucción*
instrument: *instrumento*
insufficiency: *insuficiencia*
insufficient: *insuficiente*
insular (v.): *insular*
insulator: *aislador*

insulin: *insulina*
insult: *apóstrofe, insulto*
insulting: *afrentoso*
insurance company: *compañia de seguro*
insurance policy: *póliza de seguro*
insurance: *seguro*
insurance; hospitalization: *seguro de hospitalización*
insurrection: *insurrección*
intact: *intacto*
intellectualism: *intelectualismo*
intelligence: *inteligencia*
intelligent: *inteligente*
intend to (v.): *pensar (+ infinitive)*
intense: *intenso*
intensify (v.): *avivar*
intensity: *intensidad*
intensive care: *cuidado intensivo, terapéutica intensiva*
intensive care unit: *unidad de cuidados intensivos;*
intention: *intención*
interaction: *interacción*
interest (v.): *interesar*
interest: *interés, interesar, rédito*
interested: *interesado*
interesting: *interesante*
interfere: *inmiscuirse*
interference: *injerencia, interferencia*
intermediate: *intermedio*
intermission: *recreación*
intermittent: *intermitente*
intern (v.): *internar*
intern; physician: *interno*
international: *internacional*
interpose (v.): *interponer*
interpret (v.): *interpretar*
interpretation: *interpretación*
interrogation: *interrogación*
interruption: *interrupción*
intersection: *intersección*
interval: *interval*
interview: *entrevista, entrevistar, interviú*
intestine: *intestino*
intimacy: *intimidad*
intimate (v.): *intimar*
intimate: *íntimo*
into: *en*
intoxicated: *borracho*
intoxication: *intoxicación*
intrauterine device (IUD): *aparato intrauterino*

intrauterine: *intrauterino*
intravenous injection: *inyección intravenosa*
intravenous: *intravenoso*
intravenous pyelogram: *pielograma intravenoso*
intrigue: *intriga*
introduce (v.): *innovar, introducir*
introduction: *introducción*
intuition: *intuición*
invade (v.): *invadir*
invariable: *invariable*
invasion: *invasión*
invent (v.): *discurrir, inventar*
invention: *invención*
inventor: *inventor*
inverse: *inverso*
invest (v.): *invertir*
investigate (v.): *investigar*
investigation: *investigación*
invisibility: *invisibilidad*
invitation: *convite, invitacion*
invite (v.): *convidar*
invoice (v.): *facturar*
invoke (v.): *invocar*
involve (v.): *enzarzar*
iodine: *yodo*
ireland: *irlanda*
iris: *irid, lirio*
iritis: *iritis*
iron; the mineral: *hierro*
iron; for clothes: *plancha*
irony: *ironía*
irregular (v.): *irregular*
irregular: *informal*
irreproachable: *intachable*
irresistible: *irresistible*
irresponsable: *irresponsable*
irrigator: *regador*
irritabitity: *irritabilidad*
irritable: *enojadizo, irritable*
irritate (v.): *irritar, exacerbar*
irritated: *irritado*
irritation: *irritación*
irruption: *irrupción*
is it: *es, esta*
is there; are there: *¿hay?*
island: *isla, isleño*
isolate (v.): *aislar, apartar*
isreal: *isreal*
isreali: *israelí*
it: *él, ella, ello*
it isn't: *no es, no esta*
it's: *su, suyo*

italic: *cursivo*
italy: *italia*
itch: *picazón, comezón, prurito*
itinerary: *itinerario*
IUD: *aparato intrauterino, dispositivo intrauterino*
ivory: *marfil*

J

jack: *boliche, gato*
jacket: *chaqueta*
jam; for toast: *mermelada*
jamaica: *jamaica*
january: *enero*
jar: *jarra, tarro*
jargon: *jerigonza*
jaundice: *piel amarilla "yellow skin", ictericia*
jaw: *mandíbula, quijada*
jaws: *fauces*
jealous: *celoso*
jean: *dril*
jelly: *jalea, gelatina*
jellyfish: *medusa*
jet: *jet (avion)*
jewel: *joya, alhaja*
jeweler: *joyero*
jewelry: *joyería*
jewish: *judío*
job: *empleo*
join (v.): *empalmar*
joint: *articulación, conjunto, coyuntura*
joke (v.): *bromear*
jones: *adicción de basquetbol*
jostle (v.): *codear*
journalism: *periodismo*
journey: *jornada, recorrido, viaje*
joy: *alborozo, gozo, júbilo*
joyous: *gozoso*
judge: *juez*
juggler: *malabarista*
juice: *jugo*
juice; grapefruit: *jugo de toronja*
juice; orange: *jugo de china, jugo de naranja*
juice; tomato: *jugo de tomate*
juicy: *jugoso*
july: *julio*
jump (v.): *saltar*
junction: *encrucijada, juntura*
june: *junio*

jungle: *selva*
junk: *basura*
jurist: *jurista*
juror: *jurado*
just: *justiciero, justo, sólo*
justice: *justicia*

K

kangaroo: *canguro*
keen: *aficionado*
keep: *guardar, preservar, quedarse con*
kerosene: *korosena, aceite de lámpara*
key: *clave, llave*
keyboard: *teclado*
kick (v.): *patear*
kid; baby goat: *cabrito*
kid; young child: *niño*
kidney disease: *enfermedad de los riñones*
kidney stone (slang): *piedra nefrítica, mal de piedra "stone sickness," piedra en el riñón "kidney rock"*
kidney stone: *cálculo en el riñón*
kidneys: *riñónes*
kill (v.): *matar*
killer: *matador*
killing: *matador*
kilo: *kilo*
kilometer: *kilómetro*
kind (friendly): *amable*
kind (type): *tipo, clase de*
kind, gentle: *gentil*
kindergarten: *kínder (slang), parvulario, escuela de párvulos*
king: *rey*
kingdom: *reino*
kiss (v.): *besar*
kitchen: *cocina*
kleptomaniac: *cleptómano*
knead (v.): *amasar*
knee bone: *hueso de la rodilla, rótula*
knee: *rodillas*
knife: *cuchillo, machete*
knock down (v.): *noquear*
knock in (v.): *clavar*
knot (v.): *anudar*
knot: *nudo, lazo*
know (v.): *conocer, saber*
knowledge: *conocimiento*
knuckle: *nudillo, artejo*

L

label (v.): *rotular*
label: *etiqueta*
labor pains: *dolores del parto, "los dolores"*
labor; with a child: *parto*
labor; work: *labor*
laboratory: *laboratorio*
laborer: *jornalero, trabajador, labrador*
lace: *encaje*
laceration: *laceración*
lack (v.): *carecer*
lacrimation: *lágrimación, lágrimas*
lactation: *lactación*
lad: *chaval*
ladies' room: *damas*
ladle: *cucharón*
lady: *señora, dama*
lagoon: *laguna*
lake: *lago*
lamb: *cordero*
lame: *cojo*
lament: *lamento*
lamp: *lámpara*
lance: *lanza, asta*
land: *aterrizar, desembarcarse, terreno*
landing: *meseta, rellano*
landlord: *arrendador*
language: *idioma, lengua*
laparoscopy: *laparoscopia*
laparotomy: *laparotomía*
lapse (v.): *caducar*
larch: *alerce*
lard: *manteca*
large: *grande, caudaloso*
larva: *larva*
laryngitis: *laringitis*
larynx: *laringe*
lash: *latigazo*
last night: *anoche*
last year: *el año pasado*
last; enture (v.): *durar*
last; final: *último*
late: *tarde, retrasado*
lately: *últimamente*
latent: *latente*
later: *después, luego, más tarde*
latitude: *latitud*
laudable: *laudable*

laugh (at) (v.): *reírse (de)*
laugh: *carcajada*
launch: *chalupa*
laundry: *lavandería*
laurel: *laurel*
lava: *lava*
lavatory: *lavatorio*
law: *ley*
lawsuit: *litigio*
lawyer: *abogado, licenciado*
laxative: *laxante, purgante*
lay down (v.): *deponer, posar*
lay: *laico*
laziness: *pereza*
lazy: *perezoso-a, holgazán*
lead (v.): *acaudillar*
leafy: *frondoso*
leak out: *divulgarse*
lean: *ladearse*
lean on: *acomodarse en*
leap: *salto*
learn (to) (v.): *aprender (a)*
learn (v.): *aprender*
lease: *arrendar, locación*
least: *menor, mínimo, menos*
leave (v.): *dejar, salir, abandonar*
left; opposite of right: *izquierdo*
legs: *piernas*
legality: *legalidad*
legend: *leyenda*
legion: *legión*
legislate (v.): *legislar*
legitimate: *legítimo*
leisure: *desocupación, holganza, ocio*
lemon: *limón*
lemonade: *limonada*
lend (v.): *prestar*
length: *longitud*
lens: *lente*
leopard: *leopardo*
leprosy: *lepra*
lesion: *lección*
less: *menos*
lesser: *menor*
lesson: *escarmiento, lección*
let go of (v.): *soltar*
letter: *carta, jota, letra*
lettuce: *lechuga*
leukemia: *leucemia*
level (v.): *allanar, arrasar*
level: *nivelado, nivelada*
lever: *asa*
lewd: *lascivo*
lexicon: *léxico*

liar: *mentiroso*
liberty: *libertad*
library: *biblioteca, librería*
lice: *piojos*
license: *licencia*
lick (v.): *lamer, relamer*
licorice: *orozuz*
lie (v.): *mentir*
lie down/recline (v.): *acostar(se), echarse, recostarse, tenderse*
lie face down (v.): *acostarse boca abajo*
life: *vida*
lifeguard: *bañero*
lift (v.): *levantar, alzar*
ligament: *ligamento*
light (color): *claro*
light (v.): *alumbrar*
light: *luz, liviano, liviana*
light; to turn off: *apagar la luz*
light; to turn on: *encender la luz*
lighter; of cigarettes: *encendedor*
lighthouse: *faro*
likable: *simpático*
like, such: *como tal*
like; similar: *como, par, cual*
like; to be pleasing to (v.): *gustar*
lilac: *lila*
lily: *mosca, nardo*
limb: *miembro*
lime: *cal*
limit (v.): *coartar, limitar*
limit: *confín, limite*
limitation: *limitación*
limited: *limitado*
limp (v.): *claudicar*
line (v.): *forrar*
line: *línea*
linen: *ropa de cama*
linguist: *lingüista*
liniment: *linimento*
link: *vínculo, enlace*
linoleum: *linóleo*
lion: *león*
lip: *labio*
lips: *labios*
lipstick: *lápiz de labios*
liquid: *liquido*
liquour: *licor*
lisp (v.): *cecear*
lisp: *ceceo*
list: *lista, nómina, repertorio*
listen (v.): *eschuchar*
literature: *literatura*

litter: *camada*
little (a few): *un poco*
little (small): *pequeño, pequeña, chicho*
live (v.): *vivir*
lively: *resalado, vital, animado*
liver disease: *enfermedad del hígado*
liver: *hígado*
living room: *sala*
living: *vivo*
load: *carga*
loan: *empréstito, prestamo*
lobby: *lobby, sala de recepción, vestíbulo, zaguán*
lobectomy: *lobectomía*
lobster: *langosta*
local: *local*
lock: *cerradura*
lock up (v.): *enjaular*
lock; padlock: *candado*
locomotion: *locomoción*
lodge (v.): *alojar*
log: *leño*
logical: *lógico*
lonely: *solitario*
long ago: *antaño*
long for (v.): *ansiar*
long: *largo*
long time: *mucho tiempo*
long-winded; tiresome: *prolijo*
look after: *encargarse de, ocuparse con*
look at (v.): *mirar*
look for (v.): *buscar*
look into (v.): *ojear*
look!: *¡mira!, asptecto*
loop: *lazo*
loose: *suelto, suelta, flojo, holgado, relajado*
loosen: *desajustarse*
lordosis: *lordosis*
lose (v.): *perder*
lose consciousness (v.): *perder el conocimiento*
lose weight (v.): *perder peso*
loss of conciousness: *perdida del conocimiento*
loss: *pérdida*
lost: *extraviado*
lot: *lote*
lotion: *loción*
lottery: *lotería*
love (v.): *amar*
love: *amor*

lover: *galán, amante*
low: *bajo*
low blood pressure: *presión baja*
low salt: *con poco sal*
low tide (v.): *bajamar*
lower (v.): *arriar*
lower the price (v.): *abaratar*
loyal: *leal*
lubricant: *lubricante*
lubricate (v.): *aceitar*
lucid: *lúcido*
luggage: *equipaje*
lukewarm: *tibio*
lull: *ileno-a*
luminary: *lumbrera*
lump: *bulto, protuberancia, chichón*
lunatic: *demente, lunatico*
lunch: *almuerzo*
lung disease: *enfermedades pulmones*
lung x-ray: *radiografía de los pulmones*
lungs: *pulmones, pulmón*
luxury: *lujo*
lye: *lejia*
lying down: *acostado*
lying: *mentira*

M

macaroni: *macarrones*
machine: *máquina*
machinist: *maquinista*
mad; angry: *enojado, furioso*
mad; insane: *loco*
madam: *senora*
madness: *demencia, locura*
magazine: *revista*
magic: *magia*
magician: *mágico*
magnet: *imán*
magnetize (v.): *magnetizar*
magnificent: *magnifico*
mahogany: *caoba*
maid: *sirvienta, doncella*
mail: *correo*
mailman: *cartero*
main: *mayor*
maintain (v.): *mantener*
maintainable: *mantenible*
maintenance: *mantenimiento*
majestic: *majestuoso*
majesty: *majestad*
majority: *mayoría*

majority of: *la mayoría de*
make (v.): *hacer, confeccionar*
make a decision (v.): *tomar una decisión*
make a fist (v.): *hacer un puño*
make an analysis (v.): *hacer un análisis*
maker: *hacedor*
making: *hechura*
malaria: *malaria, paludismo*
male: *masculino, hombre, varón, macho*
malfunction (v.): *funcionar mal*
malignancy: *malignidad*
malignant: *maligno*
mallet: *mazo*
malnutrition: *mala nutrición, desnutrición, malnutrición*
mammogram: *mamografía, rayos equis del senos*
mammography: *mamografia*
man: *hombre, señor*
manage: *apañarse*
manager: *gerente*
mandarin: *mandarín*
manger: *pesebre*
mango: *mango*
manic-depressive: *maniacodepresivo*
manner: *manera*
manner: *manera*
manners: *ademanes*
manpower: *mano de obra*
manual: *manual*
manufacture: *fabricación*
manufacturer: *fabricante*
many: *múltiple, muchos*
many; many more: *muchos más*
many; many times: *muchas veces*
many; so many: *tantos*
many; too many: *desmasiados*
map: *mapa*
maple: *arce*
marble: *canica*
march; month: *marzo*
march; on foot: *marcha*
margarine: *margarina*
marijuana: *marihuana, marijuana*
marine: *marino*
marital: *marcial*
mark (v.): *marcar*
mark: *mancha, marca*
market: *mercado*
marriage: *boda, casamiento*
married: *casado, casada*

marry (v.): *casar*
martyrdom: *martirio*
marvelous: *maravilloso*
masculine: *musculino*
mask: *antifaz, carátula, careta*
mason: *albañil*
mass: *macizo*
massacre: *masacre*
massage: *masaje*
mast: *mástil*
mastectomy: *mastectomía*
masticate (chew) (v.): *masticar*
mastication: *masticación*
mastoiditis: *mastoiditis*
masturbate (v.): *masturbar*
masturbation: *masturbación*
mat: *estera*
match; counterpart: *compañero*
match; for starting a fire: *el fósforo, cerillo*
match; game: *match*
match; partner for marriage: *partido*
mate (v.): *parear*
material: *material*
maternal: *materno*
maternity: *maternidad*
mathematician: *matemático*
matter: *asunto, cuestión, materia*
mattress: *colchón*
maximum: *máximo*
may: *mayo*
maybe: *quizá, quizás, ascaso*
mayonnaise: *mayonesa*
mayor: *alcalde*
me: *me*
meal: *comida*
mean; stingy: *agarrado, mezquino, tacaño*
means: *los medios*
meanwhile: *entretanto*
measles: *sarampión*
measles; german: *rubéola*
measure (v.): *medir*
measure: *medida*
meat: *carne*
mechanic: *mecánico*
mechanical: *mecanico*
mechanism: *mecanismo*
medal: *medalla*
medical: *médico*
medical records: *archivo clínico*
medical records department: *departamento de archivo clínico*
medical student: *estudiante de medicina*

medication: *medicación, medícinas, medicamento*
medicine: *medicina, medicamento*
mediocre: *mediano, mediocre*
medium: *mediano*
meeting: *mitín*
melamine: *melamina*
melodious: *melodioso*
melon: *melón*
melt (v.): *derretir, descuajar*
melted: *derretido*
melting: *fusión*
member: *miembro, socio*
memo: *apunte*
memoirs: *memorias*
memory: *memoria*
men: *señores, hombres*
men's room: *el servicio*
mend: *remiendo*
meningitis: *meningitis*
menopause: *menopausia*
mens' room: *caballeros*
menstruate (v.): *menstruar*
menstruation: *menstruación, regla*
mental health department: *departamento de enfermedades mentales*
mental hospital: *hospital mental*
mental illness: *enfermedades mentales*
mental: *mental*
mentally retarded: *atrasado mentalmente*
mention (v.): *mencionar*
menu: *menú, lista de comidas*
meow (v.): *maullar*
merchant: *comerciante*
mercy: *clemencia*
merge: *fundirse*
merit: *mérito*
merry christmas: *¡felices navidades!, ¡felices pascuas!*
merry: *regocijado*
mescaline: *mescalina*
mess: *revoltijo*
message: *mensaje*
metabolism: *metabolismo*
metal: *metal*
meter: *metro, contador*
method: *método*
meticulous: *meticuloso*
metritis: *metritis*
mexico: *méxico*

mickey mouse (rat): *ratón miguelito*
microbiology: *microbiología*
microphone: *micrófono*
microscope: *microscopio*
middle: *medio*
midnight: *medianoche*
midwife: *partera, comadre*
migraine: *migraña, jaqueca*
mild: *apacible*
mile: *milla*
milk: *leche*
milk of magnesia: *leche de magnesia*
milk; of cows: *leche de vaca*
milk; powder: *leche en polvo*
milk; raw: *leche fresca*
milk; skim: *leche descremada*
milk; teeth: *diente de leche*
milkmaid: *lechera*
mill: *molino*
miller: *molinero*
million: *millón*
mime: *mimo*
mimicry: *mímica*
mine: *mina*
miner: *minero*
mineral: *mineral*
mineral water: *agua mineral*
miniature: *minatura*
minimum: *mínimo*
minister: *ministro*
mint: *hierbabuena, menta*
minutes: *minutos*
miracle: *milagro*
mirage: *espejismo*
mirror: *espejo*
miscarriage: *aborto accidental*
miser: *avaro*
misfortune: *desdicha*
mislead (v.): *desorientar*
miss (v.): *errar*
miss, miss (female): *señorita, srta.*
miss; miss the target: *errar el tiro*
misses: *señora, sra.*
mist: *bruma, neblina*
mistake: *error, desacierto*
mister, mr.: *señor, sr.*
mistress: *maestra*
misty: *brumoso*
mite: *ácaro*
mix (v.): *entreverar*
mix up (v.): *mezclar*
mixed: *mixto*
mixer: *batidora*
mixture: *mezcla*

moan: *gemido*
mob: *chusma*
mobile: *móvil*
mobility: *movilidad*
mock (v.): *escarnecer, mofar*
model: *maqueta, modelo*
moderate: *moderado*
moderation: *moderación*
modern: *moderno*
modest: *modesto, púdico, recatado*
modify (v.): *modificar*
moist: *húmedo*
molar: *muela*
moldy: *mohoso*
mole; on the skin: *lunar*
mole; small gound animal: *topo*
moment: *momento*
monday: *lunes*
money: *dinero, plata*
mongolism: *mongolismo*
monitor: *monitores*
monk: *monje*
mononucleosis: *mononucleosis*
monster: *monstruo*
monstrous: *monstruoso*
month: *mes*
monthly: *mensual*
months: *meses*
monument: *monumento*
moo (v.): *mugir*
moon: *luna*
moral: *moral*
morality: *moralidad*
morally: *moraimente*
morbid: *morboso*
more: *más*
more or less: *más o menos*
morning: *en la mañana, mañana, matinal*
morning sickness: *náuseas del embarazo, vómitos del embarazo*
moroccan: *morroquí*
morocco: *marruecos*
mortal: *mortal*
mortification: *mortificación*
mosque: *mezquita*
mosquito: *mosquito*
moss: *musgo*
most: *la major parte*
mother: *madre, mamá*
mother-in-law: *suegra*
motion: *moción*
motive: *motivo*
motor: *motor*

mount: *cabalgadura*
mountain: *montaña, sierra*
mourning: *luto*
mouse: *ratón*
moustache: *bigote*
mouth: *boca*
mouth; roof of the: *cielo de la boca*
movable: *movible*
move back (v.): *cejar, regresar*
move: *cambiarse, moverse*
move down; lower (v.): *bajar*
move forward (v.): *adelantar*
movement: *movimiento*
movie theater: *cine*
mow (v.): *guadañar*
much: *mucho*
mucous: *mucoso*
mud: *barro, cieno, fango*
muffle (v.): *embozar*
muffler: *rebozo*
mule: *mula*
multicolored: *multicolor*
multiple sclerosis: *esclerosis múltiple*
mum: *mamá*
mumble (v.): *mascullar*
mummy: *momia*
mumps: *paperas*
murder: *asesinar, asesinato*
murderer: *asesino*
murmur: *sopla, murmullo, rumoreo*
muscles: *músculos*
muscular dystrophy: *distrofia muscular*
museum: *museo*
mushroom: *champiñón, hongo, seta*
music: *música*
musical: *músico*
musician: *músico*
mustache: *bigote*
mustard: *mostaza*
mute: *mudo*
mutilate (v.): *mutilar*
mutual: *mutuo*
muzzle (v.): *amardazar*
my: *mi*
myalgia: *dolor de músculo*
myocardial infart: *infarto miocardíaco*
myocarditis: *miocarditis*
myopia: *miopia*
myrtle: *arrayán*
myself: *me, mí*
mysterious: *misterioso*
mystery: *misterio*

mysticism: *misticismo*
myth: *mito*

N

n.p.o.; nothing by mouth: *nada para la boca*
nag: *rocín*
nail; fingernail: *uña*
nail; for wood: *clavo*
name (v.): *apellidar, nombrar*
name: *nombre*
name; first: *nombre, primero nombre*
name; last: *apellido*
nap (v.): *dormir en la día, tomar una siesta*
nap: *lanilla, siesta*
nape: *nuca*
napkin: *servilleta*
narcotic: *narcótico*
narrate (v.): *narrar*
narration: *narración*
narrator: *narrador*
narrow (v.): *estrechar*
narrow: *angosto, angosta, estrecha*
nasal congestion: *congestión nasal*
nation: *nación*
nationality: *nacionalidad*
native: *nativo, autóctono*
natural: *natural*
naturally: *naturalmente*
naturalness: *naturalidad*
nature: *naturalmente*
naughty: *revoltoso*
nausea: *náusea*
nausea; severe nausea with vomiting: *basca*
nauseating; smelly: *apesta*
navel; umbilicus: *ombligo*
navigation: *navegación*
near: *cerca, cercana, allegado*
neat: *apuesto, arreglado*
necessary: *necesario*
necessity: *necesidad*
neck: *cuello*
necklace: *collar, gargantilla*
necrosis: *necrosis*
need (v.): *necesitar, precisar*
need: *necesidad*
needle (hypodermic): *aguja hipodermica*
needle: *aguja*
needy: *apurado*

negation: *negación*
negligence: *negligencia, descuido*
neighbor: *vecino, prójimo*
neither: *ninguno, tampoco, ni*
neonatology: *neonatología*
nephew: *sobrino*
nephritis: *nefritis*
nerves: *nervios*
nervous: *agitado, nervioso, nervudo*
nervous shock: *choque nervioso*
nervous system: *sistema nervioso*
nervousness: *nervioso, nerviosidad*
nest: *nido, anidar*
net: *neto, red*
nettle: *ortiga*
neuralgia: *neuralgia*
neurasthenia: *neurastenia*
neurologist: *neurólogo-a*
neurology: *neurología*
neutral: *neutral*
neutrality: *neutralidad*
neutralize (v.): *neutralizar*
never: *nunca*
nevertheless: *sin embargo*
new: *naciente, nuevo*
newspaper: *periódico, diario*
next day: *proximo día*
next: *próximo, contiguo*
nice: *delicado, sutil, fino, majo*
niche: *nicho*
nickel; metal: *níquel*
nickname: *apodar, mote*
niece: *sobrina*
night: *noche*
night: *noche*
night sweats: *sudores en la noche*
nightingale: *ruiseñor*
nightmare: *pesadilla*
nine: *nueve*
nineteen: *dieci-nueve*
ninth: *noveno*
ninty: *noventa*
nipple on bottle: *pezón de biberón*
nipple: *pezón, tetero*
nitrate: *nitrato*
nitrogen: *nitrógeno*
no admittance: *entrada prohibida*
no: *no*
no one: *nadie*
no smoking: *no fumar*
noble: *noble*
nobody: *nadie*
nocturia: *orinas durante la noche "urinate during the night," nicturia*

noise: *ruido, estrépito*
noisy: *chillón*
nomad: *nómada*
nomenclature: *nomenclatura*
none: *ninguno, nada*
noodle: *tallarín*
noon: *medio dias, mediodía*
nor: *ni, tampoco*
normal: *normal*
normalize (v.): *normalizar*
north: *norte*
norway: *noruega*
nose: *nariz*
nosebleed: *salirle sangre de la nariz, la hemorragia nasal*
nostrils: *fosas nasales, narices, ventana de la nariz*
not at all; you're welcome: *no hay de qué*
not at all: *no del todo*
not: *no*
not yet: *no todavía, todavía no*
notable: *notable, notabilidad*
note: *anotación*
note down (v.): *anotar*
nothing by mouth (npo): *nada para la boca*
nothing: *nada*
notice; note (v.): *notar, advertir*
notify (v.): *notificar, noticiar*
notion: *noción*
nourishing: *alimenticio*
novel: *novedoso*
november: *noviembre*
novice: *novicio*
now: *ahora, áca, actualmente*
nowadays: *hoy día*
noxious: *nocivo*
nozzle: *boquilla*
nude: *desnudo*
nuisance: *chinche*
numb (v.): *entumecer*
numb: *dormido.*
number: *número, cifra*
numbness: *adormecimiento*
numeral: *cifra*
numerous: *numerosos*
nun: *monja*
nuncio: *nuncio*
nurse: *enfermero-a*
nurse; from breast (v.): *dar pecho, dar de mamar*
nurse; wet nurse: *nodriza*
nursemaid: *niñera*

nursery: *cunero*
nursing: *enfermería*
nut: *nuez*
nutmeg: *nuez moscada*
nutrition: *nutrición*
nylon: *nylon*

O

o.r. room: *sala de operaciónes*
o.r. table: *mesa de operaciónes*
oak: *roble*
oar: *remo*
oasis: *oasis*
oath: *juramento*
oats: *avena*
obedience: *obediencia*
obese: *obeso*
obesity: *obesidad*
obey (v.): *obedecer*
object: *objectar, objecto, oponerse*
oblique: *oblicuo*
obnoxious: *odioso-a*
obscene: *obsceno*
observable: *observable*
observation: *observación*
observe (v.): *observar, otear*
obsession: *obsesión*
obsession: *obsesión*
obstetrician: *obstétrico-a, partero*
obstetrics: *obstetricia*
obstruct (v.): *obstruir*
obstruction: *obstrucción*
obtain (v.): *conseguir*
obtainable: *obtenible*
obvious: *evidente, obvio*
obviously: *obviamente*
occultism: *ocultismo*
occupation: *ocupación*
occupied: *ocupado*
occur (v.): *ocurrir*
occur: *celebrarse*
october: *octubre*
odd: *impar*
odontology: *odontologia*
of course: *por supuesto*
of: *de*
offend (v.): *ofender*
offer (v.): *ofrecer*
office: *consultorio, oficina*
official: *oficial*
often: *a menudo*
oil: *aceite*

oil lamp: *candil*
oily: *aceitoso*
ointment: *ungüento, unto, pomada*
old: *anciano, viejo*
older: *mayor*
oldest: *el mayor, la mayor*
olive: *olivo*
omelette: *tortilla*
omen: *augurio*
ominous: *ominoso*
omission: *omisión*
omit (v.): *omitir*
on (upon, over): *sobre*
on: *en, encima de, sobre*
on foot: *a pie*
on one's back (face up): *boca arriba*
on the edge of: *al borde de*
on time: *a tiempo*
on top of: *encima de*
one more: *uno mas, una mas*
one time: *una vez*
one: *uno, un*
oneself: *se*
onion: *cebolla*
only: *solamente, únicamente*
opal: *ópalo*
opaque: *opaco*
open (no closed): *abierto*
open (v.): *abrir*
open up: *abrirse*
operable: *operable*
operate (v.): *operar, accionar*
operating room: *sala de operaciones*
operation: *operación*
ophthalmologist: *oftalmólogo-a*
ophthalmology: *oftalmologia*
ophthalmoscope: *oftalmoscopio*
opinion: *dictamen*
opinion: *opinión*
opportunity: *oportunidad*
oppose (v.): *contrariar, impugnar*
opposite: *enfrente, opuesto*
oppress (v.): *oprimir*
opt for: *optar a*
optician: *óptico*
optimism: *optimismo*
option: *opción*
optometrist: *optometrista*
optometry: *optometria*
or: *o, ó*
oral lesions: *fuegos en la boca*
oral: *oral*
oral polio vaccine: *vacuna oral contra el polio, las gotas de polio*

orange: *anaranjado, naranja*
orange juice: *jugo de naranja*
orbit: *órbita*
orchard: *huerto*
orchestra: *orquesta*
orchid: *orquídea*
order; harmony: *orden*
order; request: *orden*
order: *consigna*
order; command (v.): *mandar*
orderly: *asistente*
ordinary: *ordinario*
organ: *órgano*
organism: *organismo*
organs; genital: *órganos genitales*
orgy: *orgía*
orphan: *huérfano*
orthodontics: *ortodontología*
orthopedic: *ortopédico*
orthopedics department:
  departamento de ortopedia
orthopedist: *ortopédico-a*
osteomyelitis: *osteomielitis*
osteopathy: *osteopatía*
other: *otro*
others: *otros*
otitis: *otitis*
otorhinolaryngology: *otorrino-
  laringología*
ouch!: *¡ay!*
ounce: *onza*
our: *nuestro*
outline: *contorno*
outpatient clinic: *clínica paciente-
  ambulante*
outpatient: *paciente-ambulante*
outrage: *desaguisado*
outside; not inside: *externo*
outside; outdoors: *afuera, fuera*
outside of: *fuera de*
oval: *oval*
ovary: *ovario*
ovation: *ovación*
oven: *horno*
over: *encima, sobre (above)*
overalls: *overol*
overcoat: *abrigo*
overdose: *dosis excesiva, sobredosis*
overdue: *atrasado*
overflow: *desbordarse*
ow, ow, ow!: *¡ay, ay, ay!*
owe (v.): *deber, adeudar*
owl: *búho*
owner: *amo, dueño*

ox: *buey*
oxygen: *oxígeno*
oyster: *ostra*

P

p.c.; after meals: *después de las
  comidas*
p.o.; by mouth: *por la boca*
p.r.; by rectum: *en el recto*
pacemaker: *marcapaso*
pacific: *pacífico*
pacity (v.): *apaciguar*
pack (v.): *atestar*
package: *bulto, paquete*
packet: *paquete*
pact: *pacto*
pad (v.): *acolchar, rellenar*
padlock: *candado*
page: *página*
paid: *asalariado, pagado, pagada*
pail: *balde*
pain: *dolor, pena*
pain; boring: *dolor penetrante*
pain; burning: *dolor que quema*
pain; continuous: *dolor continuo*
pain; cramping: *dolor calambre*
pain; deep: *dolor hondo*
pain; dull: *dolor sordo*
pain; emotional: *pena*
pain; gripping: *dolor resgante*
pain; heavy: *dolor pesado*
pain; intense: *dolor intensivo*
pain; intermittent: *dolor intermitente*
pain; labor: *dolor del parto*
pain; light: *dolor ligero*
pain; moderate: *dolor moderado*
pain; physical: *dolor*
pain; pressure: *dolor con presión*
pain; referred: *dolor referido*
pain; ripping: *dolor rasgante*
pain; severe: *dolor severo, fuertes*
pain; sharp: *dolor agudo*
pain; shooting: *dolor punzante*
pain; tearing: *dolor desgarrante*
pain; that moves: *dolor que se mueve*
pain; throbbing: *dolor pulsante*
pain; tightness: *dolor tirantez*
painful: *penoso*
paint (v.): *pintar*
paint thinner: *desolvente de pintura*
painter: *pintor*
painting: *pintura*

pair (v.): *parear*
pair: *par*
pair; a pair of: *un par de*
pajamas: *pijamas*
palace: *palacio*
palate (v.): *paladar*
pale: *escuálido, pálido*
palm of the hand: *palma de la mano*
palm: *palma*
palm tree: *palma*
palpate (v.): *palpar*
palpitation (v.): *palpitar*
palpitation: *palpitación*
palsy: *parálisis*
palsy; cerebral: *parálisis cerebral*
pamper (v.): *mimar*
pamphlet: *folleto*
pan: *olla*
pancreas: *páncreas*
pancreatitis: *pancreatitis*
panda: *panda*
panel: *panel*
panic: *pánico*
pant; breathing (v.): *jadear*
panther: *pantera*
panties: *bragas*
panting: *jadeante*
papaya: *papaya*
paper (v.): *empapelar*
paper: *papel*
paper; paper clip: *clip*
paper; toilet paper: *papel higiénico*
parachute: *paracaídas*
parade (v.): *desfilar*
paradise: *paraíso*
paragraph: *párrafo*
parallel bars: *barras paralelas*
paralysis: *parálisis*
paralysis; cerebral: *parálisis cerebral*
paralysis; facial: *parálisis facial*
paralytic: *paralítico*
paralyze (v.): *paralizar*
paralyzed: *paralizado*
paramedic: *paramédico*
parasitology: *parasitología*
parasthesias: *sensaciones inusuales en su piel "unusual sensations in your skin"*
parcel: *embalar*
pardon (v.): *perdonar, agraciar*
parents: *los padres, progenitores*
paresis: *paresis*
park (v.): *parquear, estacionar*
parking: *estacionamiento*

parking; parking meter: *parquímetro*
parkinson's disease: *enfermedad de parkinson*
parliament: *parlamento*
parody: *parodia*
parotitis: *parotiditis, parotitis*
parrot: *loro, papagayo*
parsley: *perejil*
part: *parte*
partial denture: *dentadura parcial*
partial: *parcial*
partiality: *parcialidad*
participate (v.): *participar*
particular: *particular*
partition: *particion*
partly: *en parte*
party: *fiesta*
pass (v.): *pasar*
pass: *boleta*
passable: *pasable*
passenger: *pasajero*
passing: *pasajero*
passion: *pasión*
passive: *pasivo*
passport: *pasaporte*
past: *pasado*
paste: *empastar, pasta*
pastry shop: *pasteleria*
patch: *parche*
patella: *hueso de la rodilla, rótula*
paternal: *paterno*
path: *sendero*
pathology: *patología*
patience: *paciencia*
patient: *paciente*
patio: *patio*
patriot: *patriota*
patriotism: *patriotismo*
patrol: *patrulla*
pause: *pausa*
pave (v.): *empedrar*
pavement: *acera*
paw: *mano*
pawn (v.): *empeñar*
pay (v.): *pagar, saldar*
pay: *gajes*
payment: *pagos, abono, cobro, desembolso*
payroll: *nómina*
pea: *guisante*
peace: *paz*
peach: *durazno, melocotón*
peak: *apogeo, pico*
peal: *campanada*

peanut butter: *crema de cacahuete*
pear: *pera*
pear tree: *peral*
pearl: *perla*
peasant: *campesino*
peck (v.): *picotear*
peddler: *comerciante ambulante,*
  buhonero
pedestrian: *peatón*
pediatrician: *pediatra*
pediatrics department: *departamento*
  de pediatría
pediatrics: *pediatría*
peel: *cáscara, pellejo*
peel off: *pelarse*
peg: *clavija*
pelvis: *pelvis, cadera*
pen: *pluma*
penal: *penal*
pencil: *lápiz*
penetrate (v.): *penetrar*
penetrating: *penetrante*
penguin: *pingüino*
penicillin: *penicilina*
penis: *pene, miembro*
pension: *retiro, pension*
people: *gente*
pepper: *pimienta*
peptic ulcer: *úlcera peptica*
perceive (v.): *percibir*
perception: *percepción*
perfect: *perfecto, perfecta*
perforate (v.): *perforar*
perform (v.): *actuar*
perfumed: *perfumado-a*
perhaps: *quizás, tel vez, acaso*
pericarditis: *pericarditis*
period: *periodo, época*
period; menstrual: *regla,*
  menstruación
periodic: *periódico*
peritonitis: *peritonitis*
permanence: *permanencia*
permanent: *permanente*
permission: *permiso*
permit (v.): *permitir*
persecute (v.): *perseguir*
persist (v.): *persistir*
person: *persona*
personnel: *personal*
perspire; sweat (v.): *sudar,*
  transpirar
persuade (v.): *convencer, persuadir*
pertinent: *pertinente*

pertussis: *tos convulsiva*
pervert (v.): *pervertir*
pessimism: *pesimismo*
pest: *alimaña*
petroleum jelly: *jalea de petróleo,*
  vacelina
pharmacist: *farmacéutico*
pharmacology: *farmacologia*
pharmacy: *farmacia, botica*
phase: *fase*
phenomenon: *fenómeno*
phlebitis: *flebitis*
phlegm: *flema*
phobia: *fobia*
photo: *foto*
photograph (v.): *fotografiar*
phthisis: *tisis*
physical exam: *reconocimiento*
  médico
physical: *físico*
physical therapist: *terapista físico*
physical therapy: *fisioterapia, terapia*
  física
physician: *médico*
pianist: *pianista*
piano: *piano*
pick: *pico*
pick up (v.): *recoger, apañar*
picker (of crops): *piscador*
pickle: *pepinillo, salmuera*
pickpocket: *caco*
picture; painting: *cuadro*
picture; photograph: *foto*
pie: *pastel*
piece: *pedazo*
pier: *embaracadero*
pierce (v.): *atravesar*
pig: *cerdo*
pigtail: *coleta*
pile: *hacina*
piles: *almorranas*
pilgrim: *romero*
pill: *pastilla, píldora*
pillow: *almohada*
pillowcase: *funda*
pilot: *piloto*
pimple: *espinilla, grano, barro*
pin (v.): *alfiler*
pincers: *pinza*
pinch (v.): *pellizcar*
pine: *pino*
pineapple: *piña*
pink: *rosado, rosa, rosáceo*
pioneer: *pionero*

pipe: *tubo*
pistol: *pistola*
piston: *pistón*
pit: *hoya, platea*
pitch: *brea*
pitcher: *cántaro*
pity: *lástima, compadecerse*
placard: *pancarta*
placate (v.): *aplacar*
place (v.): *lugar, colocar*
placid: *plácido*
plague: *peste*
plaintiff: *actor*
plan: *designio*
planet: *planeta*
plant (v.): *plantar*
plant: *planta*
planter: *plantador, sembrador*
plasterer: *emplastador*
plastic: *plástico*
plate: *plato, placa, chapa*
platinum: *platino*
play (v.): *jugar*
player: *jugador*
playful: *juguetón, juguetona*
pleasant: *agradable*
please (v.): *agradar*
please; at end of a sentence: *...por favor*
please; at start of a sentence: *favor de...*
pleasure: *gusto, placer*
pledge: *arras*
plenty: *completamente*
pleurisy: *pleuresía*
plug: *enchufe*
plug in (v.): *enchufar*
plum: *ciruela*
plumber: *plomero*
plunge (v.): *sumir*
plural: *plural*
pneumonia: *pulmonía*
pocket: *bolsillo*
poem: *poema*
point at; point to: *apunta*
point: *punto, punta*
poison (v.): *envenenar*
poison: *ponzoña, veneno*
poke (v.): *atizar*
pole: *percha*
police: *policía, policíaco*
policeman: *policía*
policy; insurance: *póliza de seguro*
polio: *poliomielitis*

polio vaccine; oral: *vacuna oral contra el polio, las gotas de polio*
poliomyelitis: *poliomielitis*
polish (v.): *acicalar*
politeness: *cortesía*
pollution: *polución*
polycythemia: *policitemia*
polydypsia: *sed, sediento todo el tiempo "thirsty all the time"*
polyp: *pólipo*
polyuria: *orinas con frecuencia "urinate with frequency"*
pond: *charca*
pool: *charca*
poor: *pobre, arrastrado*
pope: *pontífice*
poppy: *amapola*
popularity: *popularidad*
population: *población*
porch: *portada*
pork: *carne de puerco, puerco*
port: *puerto*
porter: *portero, cargador*
portion: *porción, lote*
portrait: *retrato*
position: *posición*
positive: *positivo*
possibility: *posibilidad*
possible: *posible*
possibly: *posiblemente*
post: *cargo, poste, correo*
postage: *franqueo*
postage stamp: *estampilla*
postcard: *postal*
poster: *cartel*
postman: *cartero*
pot: *marmita, orinal, pote*
potable: *potable*
potato: *patata, papa*
potato; baked: *papa asada*
potato; fried: *papa frita*
potency: *potencia*
potent: *potente*
potter: *alfarero*
pound: *libra*
pour (v.): *verter*
powder: *el talco*
powder; talc: *talco, polvera*
powdered milk: *leche en polvo*
powerful: *poderoso, potente*
practicable: *practicable*
practice (v.): *adiestrar, practicar*
practice (v.): *practicar*
practice: *práctica*

pray (v.): *orar, rezar*
prayer: *rezo*
preacher: *orador*
precaution: *precaución*
precede (v.): *anteceder*
precious: *precioso*
precipitate (v.): *precipitar*
predict (v.): *augurar*
prefer (v.): *preferir, anteponer*
preferable: *preferible*
preferably: *preferiblemente*
pregnancy: *embarazo*
pregnancy test: *prueba cutánea, prueba del embarazo*
pregnant: *embarazada, encinta, preñada*
preliminary: *preliminar, eliminatoria*
prenatal care: *cuidado prenatal*
preoccupation: *preocupación*
preoccupy (v.): *preocupar*
preparation: *preparación*
preparatory: *preparatorio*
prepare (v.): *aderezar, preparar*
prescribe (v.): *recetar*
prescription: *receta*
presence: *presencia*
present: *presente*
presentable: *presentable*
presentation: *presentación*
president: *presidente*
press (v.): *apretar*
press: *aprieto*
pressure: *presión, premura*
pretext: *pretexto*
pretty: *bonito, lindo*
prevent (v.): *prevenir*
prevention: *prevención*
previous: *antecedente, previo*
price: *precio, tarifa, tasa*
prick (v.): *espinar*
pride: *orgullo*
priest: *cura, sacerdote, padre*
primary: *primario*
prince: *príncipe*
principal: *principal*
print: *estampar, grabado*
printed: *estampado*
printer: *impresor*
priority: *prioridad*
prison: *calabozo*
private: *privado*
private room: *cuarto privado*
privation: *privación*
probability: *probabilidad*

probable: *probable*
problem: *problema, trastorno*
procedure: *procedimiento*
proceed (v.): *proceder*
process: *proceso*
proclaim (v.): *proclamar, pregonar*
proctology: *proctología*
prodigious: *prodigioso*
produce (v.): *producir, operar*
product: *producto*
profess (v.): *profesar*
profession: *profesión*
professionalism: *profesionalismo*
professor: *profesor, profesora*
profile: *perfil*
profit: *beneficiarse*
profoundly: *profundamente*
prognosis: *prognosis, pronostico*
program: *programa*
progress (v.): *progresar*
prohibit (v.): *prohibir*
prohibition: *prohibición*
project (v.): *proyectar, resaltar*
projection: *proyección*
prolong (v.): *prolongar*
prominence: *prominencia*
promise: *promesa*
promoter: *promotor*
promotion: *promoción*
prompt: *pronto*
pronounce (v.): *pronunciar, fallar*
proof: *probanza, prueba*
propagate (v.): *propagar*
propensity: *propensión*
proper: *debido*
property: *hacienda*
prophylactic: *profiláctico*
propose (v.): *proponer*
prostatitis: *prostatitis*
prosthesis: *prótesis*
prostration: *postración*
protect (v.): *proteger, amparar*
protection: *protección*
protein: *proteína*
protest (v.): *protestar*
protestant: *protestante*
proud: *orgulloso-a*
prove (v.): *demostrar*
provide (v.): *guarnecer, proporcionar, proveer*
provision: *provisión*
provoke (v.): *provocar*
prune: *ciruela pasa*
psoriasis: *psoriasis*

psychiatrist: *psiquiatra*
psychiatry: *psiquiatria*
psychoanalysis: *psicoanálisis*
psychologist: *psicólogo-a*
psychology: *psicología*
psychosis: *psicosis*
pub: *tasca*
public: *público*
publication: *publicación*
publish (v.): *publicar*
pudding: *pudin*
puddle: *charco*
pull (v.): *jalar, tirar (de)*
pull down (v.): *aterrar*
pull up (v.): *arrancar*
pulsation: *pulsación*
pulse: *pulso*
pump (v.): *bombear*
pumpkin: *calabaza*
punch (v.): *golpear*
punch: *golpe, pegar, bofetón*
punctuation: *puntuación*
puncture (v.): *perforar, picar, pinchar*
punish (v.): *castigar*
pupil: *alumno, pupila*
puppet: *marioneta*
puppy: *cachorro*
purchase (v.): *comprar*
purchase: *compra*
pure: *castizo*
purify (v.): *purificar*
purple: *purpura, amoratado*
purse: *bolsa*
purse: *cartera*
pursue (v.): *perseguir*
pus: *pus*
push (v.): *empujar*
push!: *¡empuje!*
put (place) (v.): *poner*
put in a cast (v.): *enyesar, poner en yeso*
put in a sling (v.): *poner en cabestrillo*
put on: *calzar, maquillarse, ponerse*
put to bed (v.): *acostar*
putty: *masilla*
pyelogram: *pielograma*
pyetitis: *pielitis*
pyorrhea: *piorrea*

Q

q.d.; one a day: *una vez por día*

q.h.s.; before going to bed: *antes de acostarse*
q.i.d.; four times a day: *cuatro veces al día*
q.o.d.; every other day: *cada otra día*
quack: *falso, charlatán, medicastro*
quail: *codorniz*
qualify: *calificar, capacitar*
quality: *cualidad*
quantity: *cantidad*
quantum: *cuántico*
quarantine: *cuarentena*
quarrel: *rencilla*
quarry: *cantera*
quart: *cuarto*
quarter: *barriada, cuarto*
quartet: *cuarteto*
quash (v.): *sofocar, reprimir*
quay: *andén*
queen bee: *abeja reina*
queen: *reina*
question (v.): *preguntar*
question: *pregunta, cuestión*
quibble (v.): *sutilizar*
quick, rapid: *presto, rápido, veloz, ágil*
quickly: *rapidamente*
quiet (v.): *aquietar*
quiet: *callado, quieto*
quill: *pluma de ave*
quinine: *quinina*
quit: *libre, descargado*
quit; stop doing (v.): *dejar*
quite: *enteramente, bastante*
quiz: *examen*
quota: *cuota*
quotation: *cita, cotización*
quote (v.): *citizar*

R

rabbit: *conejo*
rabbit warren: *gazapera*
rabies: *rabia*
race: *carrera*
rack: *estante*
radiation: *radiación*
radio: *radio*
radioactive material: *materia radioactiva*
radioactive: *radioactivo*
radioactive substance: *substancia radioactiva*

radiograph: *radiografías*
radiography: *radiografía*
radiology: *radiología*
radish: *rábano*
rag: *andranjo*
railroad: *ferrocarril*
railway: *ferrocarril*
rain (v.): *llover*
rain: *lluvia*
rainbow: *arco iris*
raincoat: *impermeable*
raise (a child) (v.): *criar*
raise (v.): *levantar*
raisin: *pasa*
rake (v.): *rastrillar*
rancher: *ranchero*
rancor: *encono*
range: *cordillera*
rape: *violación*
rape; violate (v.): *violar*
rapidly: *rapidamente*
raramente: *hambriento*
rare: *raro*
rash: *salpullido, erupción*
rash; diaper: *escaldadura, salpullido del pañal*
raspberry: *frambuesa*
rat: *rata*
rather: *antes bien, más bien*
ration: *ración*
rave (v.): *delirar*
raw milk: *leche fresca*
raw: *bozal*
reach: *alcance*
reaction: *reacción*
reaction; allergic: *reaccion alérgica*
read (v.): *leer*
reading: *lectura*
ready: *listo*
real: *real*
reality: *realidad*
really: *de veras, realmente*
rear: *zaga*
reason: *razón*
reasonable: *razonable*
receipt: *recibo*
receive (v.): *recibir*
recent: *reciente*
receptacle: *vasija*
reception room: *sala de recepción*
receptionist: *recepcionista*
recipe: *receta*
recognition: *reconocimiento*
recognize (v.): *reconocer*

recommend (v.): *recomendar*
record: *récord*
records; achives: *archivo*
recount (v.): *referir*
recover (v.): *sanar*
recover: *cobrarse*
recovery room: *sala de recuperación*
recreation: *recreación*
recruit (v.): *alistar*
rectangle: *rectángulo*
rectum: *recto, ano*
recuperate (v.): *recuperar*
recuperation: *recuperación*
red cross: *cruz roja*
red: *rojo, colorado*
redeye: *ojo rojo*
reduce (v.): *reducir*
reduction: *reducción*
reed: *carrizo*
reel (v.): *aspar*
refer (v.): *referir*
reference: *referencia*
referring: *referente*
refine (v.): *afinar*
refinement: *refinamiento*
reflection: *reflexión*
reflex hammer: *martillo de reflejos*
refraction: *refracción*
refresh (v.): *refrescar*
refrigerator: *frigorífico, nevera, refrigerador*
refuge: *refugio, burladero*
refugee: *refugiado*
refund: *reembolso*
refuse (v.): *denegar*
regent: *regente*
regiment: *regimiento*
region: *región, comarca, distrito*
regionalism: *regionalismo*
registry: *registro*
regret (v.): *lamentar*
regular: *regular*
regularity: *regularidad*
regulate (v.): *reglamentar*
regulatory: *regulatorio*
rehabilitation: *rehabilitación*
reject (v.): *descartar, desestimar, recusar*
rejoin: *restituirse a*
relapse: *recaída*
relate (v.): *relatar, relacionar*
relation: *relación*
relationship: *parentesco*
relative: *familiar, pariente*

relatively: *relativamente*
relax (v.): *relajar, aflojar*
relay: *posta*
release (v.): *largar*
relief: *desahogo*
relieve; alleviate (v.): *aliviar, relevar*
religion: *religión*
religious: *religioso*
remain (v.): *quedar*
remain here: *quedarse aquí*
remainder: *resto, recordatorio*
remedy (v.): *remediar*
remedy: *remedio*
remember (v.): *recordar*
remember: *recordarse, acordarse (de)*
removable: *removible*
removal: *alejamiento*
remove (v.): *quitar, alejar, resecar*
renew (v.): *reanuadar, renovar*
renovate (v.): *renovar*
rent (v.): *alquilar, rentar*
repair (v.): *reparar, remendar*
repeat (v.): *repetir*
repetition: *repetición*
replace (v.): *reemplazar, reponer*
reply; response: *respuesta*
report (v.): *denunciar*
represent (v.): *representar*
reproduction (v.): *reproducir*
reptile: *reptil*
republic: *república*
repugnant: *repugnante*
reputation: *reputación*
request: *petición*
require (v.): *requerir*
requirement: *requerimiento*
rescue: *libramiento, rescate*
resemble (v.): *asemejar*
resent (v.): *resentir*
resentment: *resentimiento*
reserve: *reserva*
reservoir: *reservorio*
reside (v.): *residir*
residence: *residencia*
resident: *residente*
resign (v.): *dimitir*
resin: *resina*
resist (v.): *contrastar*
resistance: *resistencia*
resistible: *resistible*
resolution: *resolución*
resolve (v.): *resolver*
resonance: *resonancia*
resort to (v.): *recurrír a*

resource: *recurso*
respect (v.): *respetar*
respectful: *respectuoso*
respiration: *respiración*
respiratory: *respiratorio*
respiratory system: *sistema respiratorio*
respire (v.): *respirar*
respond (v.): *responder*
responsibility: *responsabilidad*
responsible: *responsable*
rest (v.): *descansar*
rest area: *descanso, area de descanso*
rest: *descanso, reposo*
restaurant: *restaurán, restaurante*
rested: *descansado-a*
restless: *inquie*
restore (v.): *restaurar*
restrain (v.): *aguantar*
restrict: *restricción*
restriction: *restricción*
result (v.): *resultar*
result: *resultado, éxito*
resume (v.): *resumir*
resuscitate (v.): *resucitar*
resuscitation: *resucitación*
resuscitation; mouth to mouth: *respiración, boca a boca*
retardation: *retardación*
retention: *retención*
retinitis: *retinitis*
retire (v.): *retirar*
retirement: *jubilación*
retract (v.): *retractar*
retreat: *retirada*
return (v.): *volver, devolver*
reveal (v.): *patentizar*
revenge: *revancha*
reverse: *revés*
review (v.): *reseñar*
review: *revisarse*
revise (v.): *revisar*
revision: *revisión, repaso*
revive: *avivarse*
revolt: *motín, pronunciarse, sublevación*
revolution: *revolución*
revolutionary: *revolucionario*
revue: *revista*
reward: *albricias, recompensa*
rheumatic fever: *fiebre reumática*
rheumatic: *reumático*
rheumatism: *reumatismo, reuma*
rhinitis: *rinitis*

rhyme (v.): *rimar*
rhythm method: *método de ritmo*
rhythm: *ritmo*
rhythmic: *rítmico*
rib: *costilla*
ribbon: *cinta, listón*
rice: *arroz*
rich: *rico*
rickets: *raquitis, raquitismo*
ride (v.): *cabalgar*
rider: *caballero*
ridicule (v.): *ridiculizar*
ridiculous: *ridiculo-a*
rifle: *fusil*
right; opposite of left: *derecha*
right; privilege: *derecho*
right now (stat): *ahora mismo*
right-hand: *derecho*
rim: *brocal*
ring (jewelery): *anillo*
ringing in ears: *zumbido*
ringworm (tinea): *tiña, empeine, enfermedad de la piel*
rinse (v.): *enjuagar*
ripe: *maduro, madura, sazonado*
ripen (v.): *madurar, sazonar*
rise: *alza, aumento*
risk (v.): *arriesgar*
risk: *riesgo*
river: *rio*
road: *carretera*
road map: *mapa itinerario*
road side: *borde de carretera*
roar: *bramido*
roast (v.): *asar, tostar*
roast: *asado*
roast beef: *rosbif*
roasted: *asado*
rob (v.): *robar*
robe: *bata*
robot: *robot*
rock: *roca, piedra*
rocky: *rocoso*
roentgenology: *roentgenología*
role: *papel, rol*
roll: *panecillo, bollo*
romantic: *romántico*
roof of the mouth: *cielo de la boca, paladar*
roof: *tejado, techo*
room: *cuarto, sala, pieza*
room; dining: *comedor*
rooster: *gallo*
root: *raíz*

rope: *soga, reata*
rosary: *rasario*
roseola: *roséola*
rot (v.): *corromper*
rotation: *rotación*
rotten: *carcomido*
rough: *áspero*
roulette: *ruleta*
round: *redondo, redonda, ronda*
route: *pasaje, rumbo, ruta*
routine: *rutina*
row: *riña, alboroto*
row; in a row: *seguidos*
rowing: *boga*
rub (v.): *estreagar*
rubbish: *basura*
rubdown: *sobada*
rubella: *rubéola*
ruby: *rubí*
rude: *grosero*
rudiment: *rudimento*
rudimentary: *rudimentario*
rug: *alfombra*
ruin (v.): *arruinar*
rule (v.): *reglar*
rule: *regla*
rumania: *rumania*
run (v.): *correr*
run away (v.): *ahuyentar*
run with (v.): *manar*
runny nose: *catarra, moquean*
rupture: *quebradura*
rural: *campesino*
rush (v.): *precipitar*
russia: *rusia*
rust (v.): *enmohecer*

S

s.t.a.t.; right now: *ahora mismo*
sabbath: *sábado "saturday"*
saccharin: *sacarina*
sack: *costal*
sacred: *sacro, sagrado*
sacrifice (v.): *sacrificar*
sad: *triste*
sadistic: *sádico*
safe: *salvo, seguro*
safely: *con seguridad*
safety pin: *seguro*
safety: *seguridad*
sag: *comba, combadura*
sail (v.): *marear, navegar*

sailor: *marinero*
saint: *san, santo*
salad dressing: *salsa, aliño*
salad: *ensalada*
sale: *venta*
saliva: *saliva*
salivation: *salivación*
salmon: *salmón*
salt: *sal*
salt water: *agua salada*
salty: *salado*
same: *mismo*
sample: *muestra*
sanatorium: *sanatorio*
sand: *arena*
sandal: *sandalia*
sandwich: *sandwich, bocadillo*
sane: *cuerdo*
sanitary napkin: *paño higiénico, servilleta sanitaria, toalla sanitaria, cotex*
sanitary: *sanitario*
sanity: *sanidad*
sapphire: *zafiro*
sardine: *sardina*
sash: *ceñidor*
satire: *libelo*
satisfaction: *satisfacción*
saturday: *sábado*
sauce: *salsa*
saucer: *platillo*
sauna: *sauna*
sausage: *chorizo, embutido*
save (v.): *ahorrar*
savings: *ahorros*
saw: *aserrar, serrucho*
saw; for wood: *sierra*
say; tell (v.): *decir*
scab: *costra*
scabies: *sarna*
scale; for weight: *escama, balanza*
scale; of a map: *escala*
scalp: *cuero cabelludo, casco*
scalpel: *escalpelo*
scan (v.): *escandir*
scandinavia: *escandinavo*
scapula: *escápula, homóplato, pateta*
scar: *cicatriz*
scare (v.): *amedrentar*
scarf: *bufanda*
scarlet fever: *escarlatina*
scene: *escena*
scented: *oloroso*
school: *escuela, liceo*

science: *ciencia*
sclerosis: *esclerosis*
sclerotitis: *esclerotitis*
scolding: *regaño*
scotland: *escocia*
scoundrel: *rufián*
scrape (v.): *raer*
scratch (oneself) : *rascarse*
scratch (v.): *arañar, rasguñar*
scratch: *raspón, rasguño*
scream: *chillido*
screen: *antipara, biombo, pantalla*
screwdriver: *destornillador*
scrotum: *escroto, la bolsa de los testículos*
scull: *espadilla*
sculpture: *escultura*
scum: *espuma, nata*
sea: *mar*
sea sick: *mareo, mareado*
seafood: *mariscos*
seal: *foca*
seamstress: *costurera*
search: *busca*
season: *estación, temporada*
seasoning: *aderezo*
seat (v.): *asentar*
seat; car seat for infant: *asiento para carro*
seated: *sentado, sentada*
seaweed: *alga*
second (v.): *secundar*
seconds: *segundos*
secret: *secreto*
secretary: *secrétario*
secretion: *secreción*
section: *seccionamiento, sección*
section; caesarean: *sección cesarea*
secure (v.): *asegurar*
security: *seguridad*
sedative: *calmante, sedante*
seduce (v.): *seducir*
see (v.): *ver*
seed (v.): *granar*
seize; to take away (v.): *apresar*
seizures: *convulsiones, ataques*
seldom: *pocas veces*
select (v.): *seleccionar*
selection: *selección*
self: *mismo, sí mismo, yo*
self-control: *cohibido, controlarse a simismo*
selfish: *egoista*
sell (v.): *vender*

seller: *vendedor*
send (v.): *enviar*
senility: *senil*
sensation: *sensación*
sense: *sentido*
sensibility: *sensibilidad*
sensible: *sensible, mirado*
sensitive: *sensible*
sensual: *sensual*
sentence: *frase, sentencia*
sentiment: *sentimiento*
separate (v.): *separar*
separated: *separado*
separation: *separación*
september: *septiembre*
septic: *séptico*
septicemia: *septicemia*
series: *serie*
serious: *grave, serio*
sermon: *prédica, sermon*
servant: *mozo, sirviente, criado*
serve (v.): *servir*
service: *servicio*
serviceable: *servible*
session: *sesión*
set; fixed: *determinado, inflexible*
set; of artificial teeth: *caja*
set; of dishes: *servicio*
set; of tennis: *partida*
set; set on (v.): *azuzar*
set; to place (v.): *poner*
settle (v.): *abonar*
seven: *siete*
seventeen: *dieci-siete*
seventy: *setenta*
several: *varios*
severe: *severo*
sew (v.): *coser*
sewer: *albañal*
sewing: *costura*
sexual relations: *relaciones (sexuales)*
sexual: *sexual*
sexy: *atractiva*
shack: *choza*
shade: *matiz*
shadow: *sombra*
shake (v.): *agitar*
sham: *simulado-a*
shame: *avergonzar, vergüenza*
shampoo: *champú*
shape (v.): *configurar, conformar*
share: *cuota*
sharecropper: *mediero*
sharp: *agudo*

shave (v.): *afeitar, rapar*
she: *ella*
sheep: *oveja*
sheet (bed): *sábana, lámina*
sheets: *sábanas*
sheik: *jeque*
shelf: *anaquel, tabla*
shell: *concha*
shellfish: *mariscos*
shelter (v.): *abrigar*
shelter: *refugio*
shepherd: *pastor, borrequero*
sheriff: *alguacil, policía*
sherry: *jerez*
shield: *escudo*
shift: *turno*
shin: *espinilla, canilla*
shine (v.): *brillar*
ship: *barco*
shipment: *embarque*
shirt: *camisa*
shiver (v.): *tiritar*
shock: *choque*
shock; frighten (v.): *susto*
shoe shiner: *limpiabotas, bolero*
shoe: *zapato*
shoemaker: *zapatero*
shoot (v.): *disparar, fusilar*
shoot: *brote*
shop: *tienda*
shop window: *vitrina*
shopkeeper: *dependiente-a*
shore: *costa, orilla*
short: *bajo*
short; brief: *corto, corta, breve*
shortcut: *atajo*
shorten (v.): *acortar*
shorts; underwear: *calzones*
shorts; pants: *pantalon corto*
shot: *balazo*
should: *deber*
shoulder blade: *escápuia, homóplato*
shoulder: *hombro*
shout: *clamor*
show (v.): *mostrar, señalar, enseñar*
show up: *asomarse*
shower: *ducha*
shrewd: *perspicaz, sagaz*
shrimp: *camarones*
shrink (v.): *contraerse, encoger*
shuffle (v.): *barajar*
shut (v.): *cerrar*
shut in (v.): *encerrar*
shutter: *postigo*

shy: *huidizo*
sick: *enfermo, malo*
sicken; take ill (v.): *enfermar*
sickle: *hoz*
sickness: *enfermedad*
side effects: *efectos secundarios*
side: *lado, bordo*
sidewalk: *acera*
sigh: *suspiro*
sight: *vista*
sightseer: *turista*
sign: *señal, asomo*
sign; make a signature (v.): *firmar*
signal (v.): *señalar*
signature: *firma*
signification: *significación*
signpost: *mojón*
silence (v.): *enmudecer, silenciar*
silence: *silencio*
silent: *taciturno, callado*
silk: *seda*
silly: *abobado*
silver: *plateado, plata*
similar: *similar*
similarity: *similaridad*
simple: *cándido, sencillo, simple*
simulate (v.): *simular*
simultaneous: *simultáneo*
sin: *pecado*
since: *desde, ya que, desde que*
sincere: *sincero-a*
sing (v.): *cantar*
singer: *cantatriz*
single: *soltero*
singular: *singular*
sinister: *siniestro*
sink: *lavamanos*
sinner: *pecador*
sinus: *seno*
sinusitis: *sinusitis*
sip (v.): *sorber*
sir: *señor, sr.*
sir, mister: *señor*
sirloin: *solomillo*
sister: *hermana*
sister-in-law: *cuñada*
sit down (v.): *sentar, asentar*
sit up (in bed) (v.): *incorporarse*
site: *emplazamiento*
situation: *situación*
sitz bath: *baño de asiento*
six: *seis*
sixteen: *dieci-séis*
sixty: *sesenta*

size: *tamaño*
skate (v.): *patinar*
skate: *patín*
skeleton: *esqueleto*
sketch: *boceto*
ski: *esquí*
skid: *resbalón*
skiing: *esquiismo*
skill: *destreza, habilidad*
skim milk: *leche descremada, leche desnatada*
skin: *piel, cuero*
skin-deep: *superficial*
skin; cracked: *grieta*
skin; discolored: *paños*
skin; dry: *piel seca*
skin; irritaion: *irritación de la piel*
skin; oily: *piel grasosa*
skin; skin test: *prueba cutánea*
skinny: *flaco, delgado*
skip: *salto*
skirt: *falda*
skull: *cráneo*
sky: *cielo*
skylight: *tragaluz*
slander: *maledicencia*
slang: *argot, modismo*
slap: *bofetada, manotazo*
slaughter (v.): *degollar*
slave: *escalvo*
sleep (v.): *dormir*
sleep: *duerme*
sleepy: *sueño*
sleeping: *durmiendo*
sleeping pill: *pildora para dormir*
sleepy: *soñoliento*
sleeve: *manga*
slender: *delgado, flaco*
slice: *lonja, raja, rebanada*
slide: *correrse*
slight: *leve*
slim: *esbelto*
sling: *cabestrillo*
slip (v.): *deslizar*
slip in: *colarse*
slippers: *zapatillas*
slogan: *lema*
slope: *cuesta*
slow: *despacio, lento, lerdo*
slowly: *despacio, lentamente*
small: *chico*
smaller: *menor*
smallpox: *viruela*
smart: *listo*

smell (v.): *oler*
smell of: *oler a*
smelling: *oliente*
smelly: *maloliente*
smile: *sonrisa, sonreírse*
smoke alarm: *alarma para humo, alarmo para incendio*
smoke; a cigarette (v.): *fumar*
smoke; as from a fire (v.): *ahumar*
smuggler: *contrabadista*
snack: *tentempié, bocadillo*
snag: *busilis*
snail: *caracol*
snake: *culebra*
sneeze (v.): *estornudar*
sneeze: *estornudo*
snore (v.): *roncar*
snore: *ronquido*
snort (v.): *bufar*
snow (v.): *nevar*
snow: *nieve*
snuff (v.): *despabilar*
so many: *tantos, tantas*
so much: *tanto*
so: *tan, así*
so that: *de modo que*
so then: *conque*
soak (v.): *calar*
soak in (v.): *penetrar*
soaked: *remojado-a*
soap (v.): *enjabonar, jabonar*
soap: *jabón*
sober: *sobrio*
sociable: *sociable*
social security: *seguridad social, seguro de social*
social services department: *departamento de servicio social*
social: *social*
socialist: *socialista*
society: *sociedad*
sociology: *sociología*
sock: *calcetín*
soda: *soda*
sofa: *sofa*
soft: *blando*
soften up (v.): *ablandar*
soil (v.): *manchar*
soldier: *soldado*
sole; of the foot: *planta del pie*
solemn: *solemne*
solemnity: *solemnidad*
solid: *sólido, denso*
solidarity: *solidaridad*

solitaty: *solitario*
soluble: *soluble*
solution: *solución*
solve (v.): *solucionar*
solvent: *solvente*
some: *algunos*
some; any: *algunos-as*
somebody: *alguien*
someone: *alguien, uno*
something: *algo*
something else: *otra cosa*
sometimes: *a veces, algunas veces*
somewhere: *algunaparte*
somnambulism: *sonambulismo*
somnolent: *soñoliento*
son: *hijo*
son-in-law: *yerno*
song: *canción*
soon: *pronto*
sooner: *más temprano, antes*
sore: *llaga, dolencia*
sore throat: *dolor de garganta*
sorry; "I'm sorry": *lo siento*
sorry; "it pains me": *me da pena*
sorry; pardon: *perdón*
soul: *alma, ánima*
sound: *sonar, sonido*
soup bowl: *sopera*
soup: *sopa, caldo*
source: *manantial*
south: *sur*
southern: *austral*
space: *cabida, espacial*
space out (v.): *distanciar*
spacious: *espacioso, amplio*
spade: *pala*
spain: *españa*
span: *palmo*
spanish: *español*
spark: *centella*
spasm: *espasmo*
spasmodic: *espasmódico*
speak (v.): *hablar*
speak: *rodeos*
special: *especial*
specialist: *especialista*
specialize (v.): *especializar*
species: *especie*
specific: *específico*
specify (v.): *especificar*
specimen: *muestra*
speech: *discurso*
speed: *velocidad*
spell (v.): *deletrear*

spend (v.): *gastar*
spent: *gastado*
sperm: *esperma*
sphere: *esfera*
spice: *especia*
spider: *araña*
spill (v.): *esparcir*
spin (v.): *girar, hilar*
spinach: *espinaca*
spine: *espinazo, la columna vertebral*
spiral: *espiral*
spirit: *brío, espíritu*
spit (v.): *escupir*
spit: *asador*
spleen: *bazo, esplíno*
splint: *tablilla*
splinter: *astilla*
split (v.): *cuartear*
spoil (v.): *ajar*
spoiled: *dañado*
sponge: *esponja*
spool: *carrete*
spoon: *cuchara*
spoonful: *cucharada*
sport: *de deporte, deportivo*
sporting: *deportivo, deportiva*
spot: *pinta, mancha*
spotting: *manchanas, coágulos*
sprain (v.): *torcer*
sprain: *torcedura, falsiado*
spread: *difundir*
spread out (v.): *desdoblar*
spring; coiled wire: *muelle*
spring; of water: *manantial*
spring; season: *primavera*
sprinkle (v.): *salpicar*
sputum: *esputo*
spy: *espía*
square: *cuadrado*
squash (v.): *aplastar*
squeak: *chirrido*
squeeze (v.): *apretar*
squid: *calamar*
squint (v.): *bizquear*
stab (v.): *apuñalar*
stab wound: *puñalada*
stability: *estabilidad*
stable; for horses: *caballeriza*
stable; static: *estable*
stage: *escenario, estadio, estapa*
stagger (v.): *tambalear*
stain: *borrón*
staircase: *escalera*
stairs: *escalera*

stairway: *escalera*
stake: *estaca*
stall (v.): *atascar*
stammer (v.): *balbucear*
stamp: *estampilla, sello, timbre*
stamp on (v.): *patear*
stand (v.): *parar, poner de pie*
stand out (v.): *destacar*
stand up (v.): *parpar*
standing: *parado, de pie*
staple: *grapa*
star: *estrella, astro*
starch: *almidón*
stare at (v.): *ojear*
start (v.): *empezar, principiar*
start; begin: *comienzo, principio*
starve (v.): *hambrear*
state: *estado*
state of health: *estado de salud*
statement: *declaración*
static: *estático*
station: *estación*
statute: *estatua*
stay awake: *desvelarse*
stay: *estadia, alojarse*
stay; remain (v.): *quedar(se)*
steak: *biftec*
steal (v.): *hurtar*
steam: *vapor*
steel: *acero*
steep: *acantilado*
stenographer: *taquígrafo*
step: *paso, escalón*
stepdaughter: *hijastra*
stepfather: *padrastro*
stepmother: *madrastra*
stepson: *hijastro*
sterility: *esterilidad*
sterilization: *esterilización*
sterilize (v.): *esterilizar*
sternum: *hueso del pecho, esternón*
stethoscope: *estetoscopio*
stew: *cocido, estofado*
stick on; stick to (v.): *pegar*
stick; as of dynamite or wood: *báculo*
stick; sting; puncture (v.): *pinchar, picar*
sticky: *pegadizo*
stiff: *tieso, entumecido*
still: *alabique, aún, todavia, quieto*
stimulant: *estimilante*
sting: *picadura*
sting; stick; puncture (v.): *pinchar,*

picar
stink (v.): *heder*
stir (v.): *remover*
stir up (v.): *amotinar*
stitch: *puntada*
stitches: *puntadas, puntos*
stock: *estirpe*
stocking: *calceta*
stoic: *estoico*
stomach ache: *cólicos, dolor de estómago*
stomach: *estómago*
stone: *cálculo, piedra*
stoop (v.): *agachar*
stop (v.): *dejar de*
stop: *alto*
store: *tienda*
stork: *cigüeña*
stormy: *borrascoso*
story (floors): *piso*
stove: *fogón*
stow (v.): *abarrotar*
strabismus: *estabismo, ojos cruz, sin control en un ojo "no control in one eye"*
straight: *recto*
straight ahead: *derecho*
strain: *torcedura*
strained: *colado*
strange: *extraño*
strap: *correa*
straw: *paja, pajita*
strawberry: *fresa*
stream: *arroyo, chorro, rambla*
street: *calle*
strength: *fortaleza, fuerza*
strengthen (v.): *esforzar*
strenuous: *estrenuo*
streptomycin: *estreptomicina*
stress: *tensión*
stretch (v.): *desentumecer*
stretcher: *camilla*
stretcher-bearer: *camillero*
strict: *estricto*
strike; hit (v.): *golpear*
string: *retahíla, ristra*
strip: *tira*
stroke: *apoplejía, derrame cerebral*
stroll (v.): *deambular*
strom: *tempestad, temporal, tormenta*
strong: *fuerte*
strychnine: *estricnina*
stubborn: *aferrado*
student: *estudiante*

studious: *estudioso*
study (v.): *estudiar*
stuff; to fill (v.): *ahitar*
stuffed nose: *nariz tupida, nariz tapada*
stumble: *traspié*
stun (v.): *atontar*
stupid: *estúpido, estúpida, bruto*
sty: *orzuelo*
style: *estilo*
stylish: *de moda*
subject: *asignatura*
sublte: *sutil*
submit (v.): *allanar*
submit to: *allanarse a*
subscription: *suscripción*
substitute: *suplente*
subtract (v.): *restar*
suburbs: *suburbios*
subway: *metro*
success: *acierto, lucimiento*
succumb (v.): *sucumbir*
such: *tal*
suck (v.): *chupar*
sudden: *brusco, repentino, súbito*
suddenly: *de repente*
suffer (v.): *sufrir*
suffer from (v.): *padecer*
sufferable: *sufrible*
sufficiency: *suficiencia*
sufficient: *bastante, suficiente*
suffocate (v.): *ahogar(se)*
suffocation: *sofocación*
sugar: *azucar*
suggest (v.): *sugerir*
suggestion: *sugestión*
suicide: *suicidio*
suitable: *aparejado*
suitcase: *maleta*
sum up: *resumen*
summary: *compendio*
summer: *verano*
summit: *cumbre*
sun: *sol*
sunburn: *quemadura de sol*
sunday: *domingo*
sunglasses: *gafas de sol*
sunny: *asoleado*
sunshade: *quitasol*
superb: *estupendo, estupenda*
superior: *superior*
supermarket: *supermercado*
superstition: *superstición*
supervisor: *superintendente,*

supervisor
supplement: *suplemento*
supply (v.): *abastecer, suministrar*
supply: *abasto*
support (v.): *apoyar*
support: *apoyo*
supportable: *soportable*
suppose (v.): *suponer*
suppository: *supositorio*
suppress (v.): *suprimir*
suppurate; exude (v.): *supurar*
suppuration: *supuración*
supreme: *soberano*
sure: *cierto, seguro*
surely: *seguramente*
surface: *superficie*
surgeon: *cirujano*
surgery: *cirugía*
surgery department: *departamento de cirugía*
surname: *apellido*
surplus: *superávit*
surprise (v.): *sorprender*
surrender: *rendición*
surround (v.): *circundar, rodear*
survival spanish; this book: *español supervivencia*
survival: *supervivencia*
survive (v.): *conservar, sobrevivir*
suspect (v.): *sospechar*
suspend (v.): *suspender*
suspictous: *sospechoso*
sutures: *puntadas, puntos*
swallow (v.): *tragar*
swallow: *trago, pasa la saliva*
swan: *cisne*
swear (v.): *jurar*
swear in (v.): *juramentar*
sweat (v.): *sudar*
sweater: *suéter*
sweating: *sudor*
sweden: *suecia*
sweep (v.): *barrer*
sweeten (v.): *endulzar*
sweets; candy: *dulces, bombóm*
swell (v.): *hinchar*
swelling: *hinchazón*
swim (v.): *bracear, nadar*
swimming pool: *piscina, pileta*
swing (v.): *balancear*
switch on (v.): *poner*
switzerland: *suiza*
swollen: *hinchado*
sword: *espada*

symbol: *sigla, símbolo*
symbolism: *simbolismo*
sympathy: *simpatía*
symptom: *síntoma, retoque*
synagogue: *sinagoga*
syndrome: *síndrome*
syndrome; down's: *minos mongolicos*
synthesis: *síntesis*
syphilis: *sífilis*
syringe: *jeringa*
syrup: *jarabe*
system: *sistema*
system; circulatory: *sistema circulatorio*
system; digestive: *sistema digestivo*
system; nervous: *sistema nervioso*
system; respiratory: *sistema respiratorio*

T

t.b. test: *prueba de tuberculina*
t.i.d.; three times a day: *tres veces al día*
table: *mesa*
tablespoon: *cuchara*
tablet: *tableta*
tachycardia: *taquicardia*
tail: *cola, rabo*
tailor: *sastre*
take (eat, drink) (v.): *tomar*
take (v.): *tomar, coger*
take a bath (v.): *bañarse*
take an x-ray (v.): *hacer una radiografía*
take charge of (v.): *encargarse de*
take down (v.): *descolgar*
take off (v.): *descalzar*
take pictures (v.): *sacar fotos*
take precautions (v.): *precaucionar(se)*
take the blood pressure (v.): *tomar la presión (de sangre)*
take the pulse (v.): *registrar el pulso*
talcum: *talco*
tale; story: *historieta*
talent: *talento*
talented: *talentoso*
talk (v.): *hablar, charlar*
talkative: *hablador, habladora*
tall: *alto, alta*
tame (v.): *amansar*

tampon: *tampón sanitario, tampón*
tangle (v.): *enredar*
tank: *tanque*
tanned: *bronceado·*
tap; faucet: *espita*
tape (adhesive): *cinta adhesiva*
tape recorder: *magnetofón*
tar: *alquitrán*
tariff: *tarifa, arancel*
tart: *golfa*
taste (v.): *catar*
tasteless: *soso*
tasty: *gustoso*
taxi: *taxi*
tea: *té*
teach (v.): *enseñar*
teacher: *profesor, maestro, instructor*
teapot: *tetera*
tear; from the eyes: *lágrima*
tear; rip (v.): *rasgar*
tearing: *lágrimación, lágrimas*
tease (v.): *embromar*
teaspoon: *cucharita, cucharada de té*
technician: *técnico*
technique: *técnica*
technology: *tecnología*
teeth: *dientes, dentadura*
teeth; to brush one's: *cepillarse los dientes*
teeth; to clean the: *limpiar los dientes*
telegram: *telegrama*
telephone call: *llamada telefónica*
telephone: *teléfono*
telescope: *telescopio*
television: *televisión, televisor, televisora*
telex: *telex*
tell (v.): *decir, referir*
temper: *berrinche*
temperament: *temperamento*
temperature: *temperatura*
temple; of the head: *sien*
temple; of worship: *templo*
temporary: *temporal*
temptation: *tentación*
ten: *diez*
tenant: *arrendatario*
tendency: *tendencia*
tender: *tierno, tierna*
tendon: *tendón*
tennis: *tenis*
tense: *tenso, tensa*
tension: *tensión*
term; as in college: *trimestre*

terminal: *ternimal*
terminal; finished: *termino, fin*
terrible: *terrible*
territory: *territorio*
terror: *terror*
terrorist: *terrorista*
test: *prueba, análisis*
test; examination: *prueba*
test; probe (v.): *probar*
testicle: *testículo*
testify (v.): *testificar*
tetanic: *tetánico*
tetanus: *tétano*
text: *texto*
thank (v.): *agradecer*
thanks a lot: *muchas gracias*
thanks: *gracias*
that; so that: *que*
that; that one: *eso*
the day after tomorrow: *pasado mañana*
the: *el*
theater: *teatral, teatro*
theft: *hurto*
them: *las*
then: *entonces, luego*
theology: *teología*
theory: *teoría*
therapeutic: *terapeútico*
therapist: *terapeuta, terapista*
therapy: *terapia, terapéutio*
there: *allá, ahí*
there are: *hay*
there isn't...: *no hay*
there is...: *hay*
therefore, so: *así que*
thermometer: *termómetro*
these: *estos, estas*
thesis: *tesis*
they: *ellas*
thick: *grueso, gruesa*
thickness: *grosor*
thief: *ladrón, ladrona*
thigh: *muslo*
thimble: *dedal*
thin (slight): *delgado, delgada*
thin: *delgado, flaco*
thing: *cosa, chisme*
things: *enseres*
think (v.): *pensar*
think about (v.): *pensar en*
thinker: *pensador*
third: *tercero*
thirst: *sed*

thirsty (v.): *tener sed*
thirsty: *sediento, con sed*
thirteen: *trece*
thirty: *treinta*
thirty-one: *treinta y uno*
this: *esto, esta, este*
this one: *esta, éste*
this thing: *esto*
thorax: *tórax*
thorn: *espina*
though: *aunque*
thought: *pensamiento*
thousand: *mil*
thrash (v.): *apalear*
thread (v.): *enhebrar*
threat: *amenaza*
three: *tres*
throat: *garganta*
thrombosis: *trombosis*
through: *a través (de)*
throw (v.): *echar, tirar*
throw away (v.): *botar*
throw up (v.): *vomitar, arrojar*
thrust; push (v.): *empujar*
thumb: *pulgar, dedo pulgar, dedo gordo*
thursday: *jueves*
thyme: *tomillo*
thyroid problems: *problemas de la tiroides*
thyroid: *tiroides*
tic: *crispatura, tremblor*
ticket window: *boletería*
ticket: *boleto*
tickle (v.): *cosquillear*
tide: *marea*
tidy: *ordenado, ordenada*
tie (v.): *atar*
tie up (v.): *atar*
tiger: *tigre*
tile: *teja*
till (v.): *arar*
tilt (v.): *ladear*
time (of day): *hora*
time: *tiempo*
times (occurances): *vez*
timid: *apocado*
tincture of iodine: *tinta de yodo*
tingling: *hormigueo*
tinsel: *oropel*
tinsmith: *hojalatero*
tiny: *chiquito*
tip (v.): *ladear*
tire; fatigue (v.): *cansar*

tired: *cansado*
tissue: *pañuelo de papel*
title: *rúbrica, título*
to: *a, para*
to him: *para él*
to the left: *a la izquierda*
to the right: *a la derecha*
to them: *para ellos*
to us: *para nosotros*
to you: *os*
toad: *sapo*
toast: *brindis*
tobacco: *tabaco*
today: *hoy*
toe: *dedo del pie*
toilet: *baño, excusado*
toilet paper: *papel higiénico*
token: *ficha*
tolerable: *tolerable*
tolerance: *tolerancia*
tolerant: *tolerante*
toll; ring (v.): *clamorear*
tomato juice: *jugo de tomate*
tomato: *tomate*
tomorrow: *mañana*
tongue depressor: *pisalengua*
tongue: *lengua*
tonight: *esta noche*
tonsillitis: *tonsilitis*
tonsils: *amígdalas, anginas*
too many: *demasiados (-as)*
too much: *demasiado*
too; also: *también*
tool: *herramienta, utensilio*
tooth decay: *carie*
tooth: *diente*
tooth; impacted: *muela impactada*
tooth; impacted wisdom: *muela del juicio impactado*
tooth; wisdom: *muela del juicio*
toothache: *dolor de muela, dientes*
toothbrush: *cepillo (para) el dientes*
toothpaste: *pasta de dientes*
top: *cima*
torment: *tormento*
torticollis: *tortícolis*
tortilla: *tortilla*
torture (v.): *atormentar, tortura*
total: *monta*
touch (v.): *tentar, tocar, palpar*
touchy: *susceptible*
tough: *hampón*
tour: *paseo*
tourism: *turismo*

tourist: *turista*
tourniquet: *torniquete*
tow: *remolque*
toward: *hacia*
towel(s): *toalla, toallitas*
town, city: *ciudad*
toxemia: *toxemia*
toxic: *tóxico*
toxin: *toxina*
toy: *juguete*
trace (v.): *calcar*
trachea: *traquea, gaznate*
tracheotomy: *traqueotomía*
track: *pista*
tractable: *tratable*
traction: *tracción*
trade (v.): *comerciar, cambiar*
tradition: *tradición*
traditional: *tradicional*
traffic: *tráfico*
tragedy: *tragedia*
tragic: *trágico*
train: *tren*
traitor: *traicionero*
tranquilizer: *calmante, tranquilizante*
transcendence: *transcendencia*
transfer (v.): *transferir*
transformation: *transformación*
transfusion (blood): *tranfusión de sangre*
transfusion: *transfusión*
transitory: *transitorio*
translate (v.): *traducir*
translator: *interpretor, traductor*
transmission: *transmisión*
transmit (v.): *transmitir*
transparency: *transparencia*
transparent: *transparente*
transportation: *transportatación*
trap (v.): *atrapar*
trap: *artimaña, trampa*
trapeze; grab bar: *barra de agarrarse*
trash: *basura*
trauma: *trauma*
travel (v.): *ir de viaje, viajar*
traveler: *viajero*
tray: *bandeja*
tray table for bed: *mesita auxiliar para la cama*
treason: *traición*
treasure: *tesoro*
treat; to heal (v.): *curar*
treatment: *tratamiento*
tree: *árbol*

tremble: *tremblor*
trembling: *temblor*
tremendous: *tremendo-a*
trepanation: *trepanación*
trial: *ensayo*
tribute: *tributo, elogio*
trichinosis: *triquinosis*
trichomonas: *tricomonas*
trick: *baza*
trickster: *burlador*
trip: *gira*
trivial: *bagatelas, trivialidades*
trouble: *apenar, molestia*
trougers; pants: *pantalones*
truck: *camión*
true: *verídico*
truly: *verdad, de veras*
trumpet: *bocina*
trunk: *baúl*
trust: *confianza*
trust in (v.): *fiar*
truth: *verdad, veras*
truthful: *verdadero*
try (v.): *probar*
try to (v.): *tratar de*
tub: *bidet, bidé*
tubal ligation: *ligadura de los tubos*
tubal: *tubárico*
tube: *tubo*
tuberculosis (t.b.): *tuberculosis*
tuberculosis test: *prueba de tuberculina*
tuesday: *martes*
tumor: *tumor*
tuna: *atún*
tunnel: *túnel*
turberculosis: *tuberculosis*
turgid: *turgente*
turkey: *pavo*
turn (v.): *doblar; torcer*
turn off; the light (v.): *apagar la luz*
turn on; the light (v.): *encender la luz*
turn over (v.): *voltear*
turn: *turno, grio*
tusk: *colmillo*
tutor: *tutor*
tweezers: *pinzas*
twelve: *doce*
twentieth: *vigésimo*
twenty: *veinte*
twenty-one: *viente y uno*
twin: *gemelo*
twinkle: *destello*
twist (v.): *torcer, retorcer*

twitch: *crispatura, tremblor*
two: *dos*
type; kind: *tipo, clase de*
typhoid fever: *fiebre tifoidea*
typhoid: *tifoidea*
typhus: *tifus*
typical: *típico*
typist: *dactilógrafo*
tyrant: *tirano*

U

u.a.; urinalysis: *análisis de orina*
u.g.i. series: *series gastrointestinal superior*
ugliness: *fealdad*
ugly: *feo, fea*
ulcer: *úlcera*
ulcerate (v.): *úlcerar*
ulceration: *úlceración*
ultrasonic machine: *máquina ultra-sónica*
ultrasound transmitter: *transmisor ultrasonido*
ultrasound: *ultrasonido*
umbilical cord: *cordón umbilical*
umbilicus: *ombligo*
umbrella: *paraguas*
unanimous: *unánime*
unbearable: *inaguantable*
unbreakable: *inquebrantable*
unbutton (v.): *desabotonar*
uncertain: *incierto*
uncle: *tío*
uncomfortable: *incomodo*
unconciousness: *insensibilidad, inconsiente*
uncontrollable: *incontrolable*
undecided: *indeciso*
under: *abajo de, bajo, debajo, so*
underneath: *abajo, debajo de*
understand (v.): *comprender*
underwear: *ropa interior*
uneducable: *ineducable*
unfortunate: *desafortunada*
unfortunately: *desafortunadamente*
unguent: *unguento*
union: *unión*
unique: *único*
unit: *unidad*
united states: *estados unidos, los*
university: *universidad*
unless: *a menos que, como no*

unmarried: *soltero*
unobservable: *inobservable*
unpleasant: *antipático*
unreasonable: *irrazonable*
unsafe: *inseguro, insegura*
unserviceable: *inservible*
unstable: *inestable*
unsupportable: *insoportable*
until: *hasta*
up: *arriba*
up to, until: *hasta*
upright: *honrado*
uproot (v.): *desarraigar*
upset: *perturbación*
upstairs: *escalera arriba*
uremia: *uremia*
urethra: *uretra*
urge on (v.): *acuciar*
urgency: *urgencia*
urgent: *urgente*
uric: *úrico*
urinal: *orinal, orina, pato*
urinalysis: *urinálisis, análisis de la orina*
urinate (v.): *orinar*
urine: *orina, orín*
urine; dark: *orin oscuro*
urine; pain: *dolor al orinar*
urology: *urología*
us: *nosostros*
usable: *usable*
use (v.): *usar*
useless: *inútil, inservible*
usher: *conserje, acomodador*
utensil: *utensilio, cachivache*
uterus: *útero*
utilize (v.): *utilizar*

V

vacant: *vacante, desocupado, vacío*
vacate (v.): *descupadar*
vacation: *vacaciones*
vaccinate (v.): *vacunar*
vaccination: *vacunación*
vaccine: *vacuna*
vacuum cleaner: *aspiradora*
vacuum: *vacío*
vagina: *vagina*
vaginal cream: *crema vaginal*
vaginitis: *vaginitis*
vagrant: *vagabundo*
vague: *borroso, vago, impreciso*

vain; conceited: *engreído, vanidoso, vano*
vale: *valle*
valet: *camarero, ayuda, paje*
valid: *valedero, valído*
valuable: *valioso, valiosa*
valuation: *aprecio*
value (v.): *avaluar*
value: *valor*
vamp: *mujer fatal*
vandalism: *vandalismo*
vanilla: *vainilla*
vanish: *disiparse*
vanity: *vanidad*
vapor: *vapor*
variable: *variable*
variation: *variación*
varicose veins: *venas varicosas*
varied: *variado*
various: *varios, varias*
varnish: *barniz*
vase: *florero*
vasectomy: *vasectomía*
vaseline®: *vaselina*
vault: *bóveda*
veal: *ternera*
vegetable: *legumbre, vegetal, verdura, hortaliza*
vehemence: *vehemencia*
vehement: *vehemente*
vehicle: *vehículo*
vein: *vena*
veins; varicose: *venas varicosas*
velvet: *terciopelo*
venereal disease: *enfermedad venérea*
venezuela: *venezuela*
ventilate (v.): *ventilar*
ventilation: *ventilación*
verbal: *verbal*
verbose: *verboso*
verdict: *fallo, veredicto*
versatility: *versatilidad*
verse: *verso*
version: *versión*
vertebral column: *columna vertebral*
vertical: *vertical*
very little: *un poquito*
very much: *muchísimo*
very: *muy*
vessel: *buque, vasija, vaso*
vest: *camiseta*
vestibule: *portal, vestíbulo*
veterinary: *veterinario*
vex (v.): *aspar*

vibration: *vibración*
vibratory: *vibratorio*
vicious: *vicioso*
victim: *víctim, víctima*
video cassette recorder: *videograbadora*
video game: *video-juego*
video tape; cassette: *cinta grabada de televisión*
vigorous: *vigoroso, vivaz*
village: *pueblo, aldea, lugareño*
vinegar: *vinagre*
violate (v.): *violar*
violation: *violación*
violence: *violencia, vehemencia*
violin: *violín*
virgin: *virgen*
virus: *virus*
viscosity: *viscosidad*
visibility: *visibilidad*
visible: *visible*
vision test: *examen de la vista*
vision: *visión, vista*
vision; blurred: *vista nublada*
vision; double: *vista doble*
visit (v.): *visitar*
visit: *visita*
visitor: *visita*
vitality: *vitalidad*
vitamin: *vitamina*
voice: *voz*
void: *oquedad*
volnerable: *vulnerable*
voltage: *voltaje*
volume: *caudal*
volunteer: *ofrescerse*
vomit (v.): *vomitar*
vomit: *vómito*
vote (v.): *votar, sufragio*
voyage: *viaje*
vulgar: *chabacano*
vulture: *buitre*

W

waddle (v.): *anadear*
wagon: *carreta*
waist: *cintura, talle*
wait (v.): *esperar*
wait for (v.): *aguardar, esperar*
waiter: *mozo, mesero, camarero*
waiting room: *sala de espera*
waitress: *camarera*

wake: *estela*
wake up: *despabilarse*
wake-up; awaken (v.): *despertar(se)*
walk (v.): *andar, caminar*
walk on (v.): *pisar*
walker: *apoyador para caminar* "helper to walk"
wall: *muralla, muro, pared*
wallet: *billetera, cartera*
wallpaper (v.): *tapizar*
wan: *macilento*
wander (v.): *errar*
want (v.): *desear, querer*
war: *guerra*
ward: *cuarto múltiple*
wardrobe: *armario*
warehouse: *bodega, almacén*
warlike: *belicoso*
warm (v.): *caldear*
warm: *caliente*
warn (v.): *advertir, amonestar, avisar*
warp: *bombearse*
wart: *verruga*
warts; genital: *verruga genital*
wash (v.): *lavar*
wash oneself: *lavarse*
washbasin: *lavabo*
washcloth: *toalla de mano, la toallita*
washerwoman: *lavandera*
washing: *colada, lavado*
wasp: *avispa*
waste: *derroche*
watch over (v.): *velar*
watch: *reloj*
watchman: *celador*
water: *agua*
water down (v.): *aguar*
water; bag of: *bolsa de agua*
water; mineral: *agua mineral*
watercress: *berro*
watering: *riego*
watermelon: *sandía*
wave: *ola*
wax: *cera*
way: *camino*
we: *nosotros*
weak: *débil*
weaken (v.): *debilitar*
weakness: *debilidad, débil*
wealth: *riqueza*
wear out (v.): *desgastar*
weather: *clima del tiempo*
weave (v.): *tejer*
wedding: *boda, matrimonio*

wedge: *calza*
wednesday: *miércoles*
weeks: *semanas*
weeping: *llanto*
weigh (v.): *pesar, abalanzar*
weigh down (v.): *agobiar*
weight change: *cambiado de peso*
weight: *peso*
weird: *raro-a*
welcome (you're): *de nada, no hay de qué*
welcome: *bienvenido-a*
welcome (v.): *acoger*
welcoming: *acogedor*
well: *bien*
well-being (v.): *bienestar*
well-earned: *bien ganado, bien ganada*
well-worn: *usado, usada*
welt: *roncha*
west: *oeste*
wet: *mojado*
wet nurse: *nodriza*
wet; moisten (v.): *mojar*
whale: *ballena*
wharf: *descargadero*
what: *¿qué?, ¿cuál?*
what date: *¿qué fecha?*
what else: *¿qué más?*
what if...: *¿y si...?*
what is that: *¿que es eso?*
wheal: *roncha*
wheat: *trigo*
wheel chair: *silla de ruedas*
wheel: *rodar, rueda*
wheeze (v.): *silbar, jadear*
when: *cuando*
where: *donde*
where?: *¿a dónde?, ¿dónde?*
which: *cuyo, cuya*
which?: *¿cuál?*
while: *mientras*
whimper (v.): *lloriquear*
whip (v.): *azotar, hostigar*
whip: *azote*
whiplash: *lastimado del cuello* "injury of the neck"
whiskey: *whiskey* (pronounced "we-ski")
whisper (v.): *cuchichear*
whistle (v.): *pitar*
white: *blanco*
whiten (v.): *blanquear*
whiteness: *albor, blancura*

who else: *¿quién más?*
who, whom: *quien, quienes*
who?, whom?: *¿quién?, ¿quiénes?*
whoever: *quienesquiera*
whole: *entero*
wholesale: *mayorista*
whooping cough: *tos ferina*
whore: *pelleja*
whose: *cuyo*
why not?: *¿cómo no?, ¿por qué no?*
why?: *¿por qué?*
wicked: *maleante*
wicker: *mimbre*
wide: *ancho*
widow: *viuda*
widower: *viudo*
width: *anchura*
wife: *esposa, mujer*
wig: *peluca*
wiggle (v.): *menear*
wild: *bravío, salvaje*
will: *talante*
wily: *capcioso*
win (v.): *ganar, captar*
wind (v.): *aspar*
window: *ventana*
windscreen: *parabrisas*
windup: *conclusión*
windy: *airoso*
wine: *vino (pronounced "vee-no")*
wing: *ala*
wink (v.): *guiñar*
winner: *ganador*
winter: *invierno*
wipe (v.): *enjugar*
wire: *alambre*
wisdom: *sabiduría*
wisdom tooth: *muela del juicio*
wise: *juicioso*
wish (v.): *querer*
wish: *deseo*
wit: *gracejo*
witch: *bruja*
with: *con*
with her: *consigo*
with him: *consigo*
with me: *conmigo*
with you: *contigo*
withdraw: *retiradar, esquivarse, quitarse*
withdrawal; remove (v.): *sacar, retirar*
within: *por dentro, dentro de*
without a doubt: *sin duda*

without salt: *sin sal*
without: *sin*
witness: *testigo*
wizard: *brujo, mago*
wolf: *lobo*
woman: *mujer*
womb: *matriz, vientre*
women: *señoras, mujeres*
women's room: *el cuarto de damas*
wonder: *maravilla*
wonderful: *estupendo*
wood: *bosque, madera*
woodworker: *ebanista*
wool: *lana*
woollen: *lanero*
woolly: *lanudo*
word: *palabra, vocablo*
work (v.): *trabajar*
work: *empleo, trabajo*
workable: *laborable*
worked: *labrado*
worker: *trabajador, obrero*
working man: *hombre trabajando, trabajor, obrer*
working woman: *mujer trabajando, trabajora, obrera*
workshop: *taller*
world: *mundo*
world; television: *telemundo*
worms: *lombrices, lombriz*
worn: *rozado*
worried: *preocupado*
worry (v.): *preocupar*
worry: *apurarse*
worse: *peor*
worsen (v.): *empeorar*
worsen: *agravarse*
worthy: *digno de*
wound (v.): *herir*
wound: *herida*
wrap (v.): *envolver*
wrap up: *rebozar, taparse*
wretch: *pelado*
wretched: *abyecto*
wriggle (v.): *serpentear*
wrinkles (-ed): *arrugas, arrugado-a*
wrist: *muñeca*
write (v.): *escribir*
writer: *escritor*
writting pad: *bloc*
wrong: *entuerto*

DICTIONARY

X

x-rated: *no recomendado, pornográfico*
x-ray department: *departamento de radiografía, departamento de rayos-x*
x-ray: *rayos-equis, radiografía, rayos x*
xenon: *xenón*
xerograph: *fotocopia instantánea en seco*

zip: *cremallera*
zone: *zona*
zoology: *zoologia*
zoom: *zumbido*
zygoma: *cigomatica*

PC: 6642

Y

yacht: *yate*
yam: *ñame, batata*
yard: *yarda*
yarn: *hilo*
yawn (v.): *bostezar*
year: *año*
yearbook: *anuario*
years: *años*
yeast: *levadura*
yell (v.): *aullar, gritar*
yellow: *amarillo*
yellow fever: *fiebre amarilla*
yes: *sí*
yesterday: *ayer*
yesterday; the day before: *anteayer*
yet todavía, aún
yet: *aún, todavía*
yogurt: *yogurt*
yoke: *yugo, yunta*
yolk; egg: *yema del huevo*
you: *os, vosotros*
you're welcome: *de nada, no hay de qué*
young: *joven, mozo, niño*
young lady: *senorita*
younger: *menor*
youngest: *el/la menor*
your: *tu, vuestro*
yours: *tuyo, vuestro*
yourself: *ti, tu mismo*
youth: *juventud, mocedad*
youthful: *juvenil*

Z

zeal: *celo*
zebra: *cebra*
zenith: *cenit*
zero: *cero*
zinc: *cinc*
zip code: *zona postal, código postal*

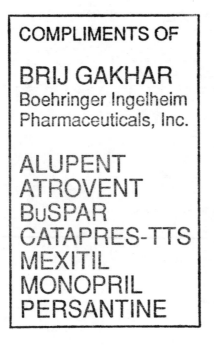

COMPLIMENTS OF

BRIJ GAKHAR
Boehringer Ingelheim
Pharmaceuticals, Inc.

ALUPENT
ATROVENT
BuSPAR
CATAPRES-TTS
MEXITIL
MONOPRIL
PERSANTINE

INDEX

METERED-DOSE INHALER INSTRUCTIONS

Atrovent® (ipratropium bromide) Inhalation Aerosol
Closed Mouth Technique

1. After removing the cap from the mouthpiece, shake the inhaler for a few seconds.

2. Hold the inhaler upright and place it in your mouth, making a seal with your lips around the inhaler. Keep your eyes closed to avoid spraying the medication into your eyes.

3. Breathe out fully, blowing out as much air as possible from your lungs.

4. Breathe in deeply and at the same time press the inhaler between your thumb and forefinger. This will force the medication from the inhaler into your throat and lungs.

5. Hold your breath for a few seconds and then remove the inhaler from your mouth and breathe normally. Wait about fifteen (15) seconds and then repeat the inhalation.

Alupent® (metaproterenol sulfate) Inhalation Aerosol

The Prescribing Information for Alupent Inhalation Aerosol recommends the closed-mouth technique, but for your information, we are also providing instructions for the open-mouth technique. Your doctor will tell you which technique to use.

Open-Mouth Technique
The steps are exactly the same, **except Step 2.** With the open-mouth technique, you place the inhaler in your mouth without fully closing your mouth around the mouthpiece.

- Try to keep the mouthpiece clean. Wash it with hot water after each use.

- Consult your doctor or nurse if you have any questions.

INSTRUCCIÓNES PARA DOSIS-MEDIDA DEL INHALADOR

Atrovent® (ipratropium bromide) Aerosol de Inhalacion
Técnica de Boca Cerrada (Closed Mouth Technique)

1. Después de quitar la tapadera de la boquilla, agitelo vigorosamente (revuelvalo) bien por unos segundos.

2. Sostenga el inhalador boca abajo y pongalo en la boca sellando con los labios el inhalador cierre los ojos para prevenir que le caga el medicamento en los ojos.

3. Sople completemente, soplando todo el aire de sus pulmones.

4. Respire profundamente al mismo tiempo (mientras inhala) qué oprime hacia abajo firmemente en el cantucho. Esto forza el medicamento dentro de su garganta y pulmones.

5. Detenga (sostenga) su aliento por unos segundos y luego retire el inhalador de la boca y respire normalmente. Espere como unos quince (15) segundos y luego repita la inhalacion.

Alupent® (metaproterenol sulfate) Aerosol de Inhalacion

La informacion prescribida para la inhalacion del aerosol Alupent recomenda la técnica de boca cerrada, pero para su informacion le damos tambien las instrucciones de la técnica de boca abierta. Su doctor le dira cual técnica usar.

Técnica de Boca Abierta (Open-Mouth Technique)

Los pasos son exactamente los mismos **con exception del paso numero 2.** Con la técnica de boca abierta usted pone el inhalador en la boca sin cerrarla completemente alrededor de la boquilla.

- Trate de mantener la boquilla limpia. Lavela con agua caliente después de cada uso.

- Consulte su médico o enfermera si tiene algunas preguntas.

TRANSDERMAL PATCH INSTRUCTIONS

Catapres-TTS® (clonidine)/Transdermal Therapeutic System
Patch Application Instructions

1. Wash hands and area where patch will be applied with soap and water. Dry thoroughly. (Select a hairless area on the upper, outer arm or chest that is free of cuts, scars, abrasions, or irritations – do not select skin folds or areas under tight garments because patch may loosen.)

2. Open the carton and remove pouch labeled Catapres-TTS.

3. Remove square, tan Catapres-TTS patch from pouch (not the white, round overlay, which does not contain medication – see below). Gently peel off clear protective backing from patch, one half at a time. Avoid touching sticky surface of patch with hands.

4. Place Catapres-TTS patch on prepared area, sticky side down. Apply firm pressure over patch to ensure good contact with skin.

5. Apply a new patch once each week to a different skin site at a convenient time on the same day of the week.

Adhesive Overlay Application Instructions

(for *optional* use as directed by your physician.)

1. The overlay does not contain medication and should be used only if required to keep the patch in place.

2. Remove round, white adhesive overlay from pouch. Remove paper backing from overlay and place overlay over Catapres-TTS patch. Apply firm pressure, especially around edges, to ensure contact with skin.

• If the Catapres-TTS patch begins to peel from the skin, the round, white adhesive overlay should be applied directly over it to ensure effectiveness for the full seven (7) days. If the Catapres-TTS patch completely falls off or loosens significantly, replace it with a new one on a different skin site.

• Even after use, a Catapres-TTS patch contains active medication that may be harmful to infants and children if accidentally applied, sucked, or swallowed. After removing the patch, fold it in half with the sticky sides together. Then carefully dispose of it out of the reach of children.

• If you experience skin irritation at the application site, or other adverse effects, contact your doctor immediately.

D

INSTRUCCIONES PARA EL PARCHE TRANSDERMAL

Catapres-TTS® (clonidine)/Transdermal Therapeutic System
Instrucciones para la Aplicacion del Parche

1. Lave con sabon y agua sus manos y el area donde el parche se va aplicar y sequese completemente. (Seleccione un lugar sin pelo en el ombro o en el pecho que no tenga cortadas, cicatrices, enmendaduras o irritaciones – no escoja plieges en la piel o areas debajo de ropa apretada porque se puede aflojar.

2. Abra le caja y saque el bolsa marcada Catapres-TTS.

3. Saque el parche cuadrado color café Catapres-TTS del bolso (no el blanco redondo que va arriba, el cual no contiene medicamento – mira abajo). Cuidadosamente quite la capa clara protectiva tracera del parche por mitades. Evite no tocar con las manos la superficie engomada del parche.

4. Ponga el parche Catapres-TTS en el area preparada, con el lado engomado para abajo. Ponga presion firme sobre el parche para asegurar buen contacto con la piel.

5. Aplique un parche nuevo una vez por semana en un lugar diferente a una hora conveniente en el mismo dia de la semana.

Instrucciones para la Aplicacion de la Tapadera Adesiva

(para el uso *opcional* como lo diriga su médico))

1. La tapadera no contiene medicamento y solo se debe de usar si se requiere para mantener el parche en su lugar.

2. Saque la tapadera adesiva blanca y redonda del bolso. Quite la capa tracera de papel del la tapadera y ponga la sobre el parche Catapres-TTS. Ponga presion firme especialmente alrededor para asegurar contacto con la piel.

- Si el parche Catapress-TTS se empieza a despegar de la piel, la tapadera adesiva blanca redonda de devede ponerse directamente sobre el parche para serciorar su eficencia por los siete (7) dias. Si el parche Catapress-TTS se despega completamente o se desprende demasiado, remplascalo (cambie) con uno nuevo en otro lugar de la piel.

- El parche Catapress-TTS contiene medicamento activo después del uso puede ser dañino a infantes y niños si se aplica, chupa o traga. Después que se remueva el parche, doblelo por la mitad con los lados engomados juntos. Tirelo cuidadosamente fuera del alcanse de los niños.

- Si le sale (experiencía) alguna irritacion en la piel en el lugar de la aplicacion o otros efectos adversos, comuniquese con su médico immediatamente.